The Happy Health Plan

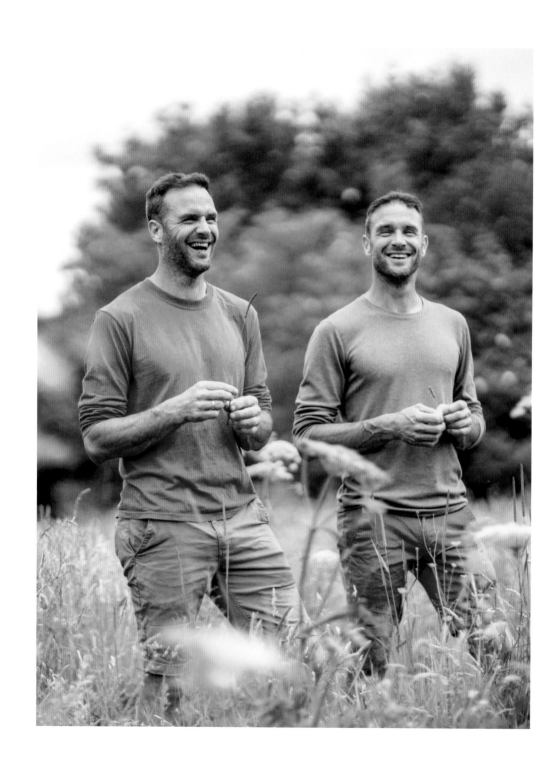

The Happy Health Plan

Simple and tasty plant-based food
to nourish your body inside and out

**David &
Stephen Flynn**

With photography by Chris Terry
Recipe photography by Maja Smend

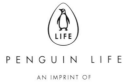

PENGUIN LIFE

AN IMPRINT OF
PENGUIN BOOKS

PENGUIN LIFE

UK | USA | Canada | Ireland | Australia
India | New Zealand | South Africa

Penguin Life is part of the Penguin Random House group of companies
whose addresses can be found at global.penguinrandomhouse.com.

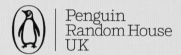

First published 2020
001

Text copyright © David and Stephen Flynn, 2020
Photographs pp. 2–105 and pp. 277–288 copyright © Chris Terry, 2020
Photographs pp. 129–271 copyright © Maja Smend, 2020

The moral right of the copyright holders has been asserted

Designed by Saffron Stocker
Colour reproduction by Altaimage Ltd
Printed in Italy by Printer Trento S.r.l.

A CIP catalogue record for this book is available from the British Library

ISBN: 978–0–241–47144–9

www.greenpenguin.co.uk

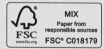

Contents

Introduction

We all want to be healthy and happy. We all want to wake up in the morning with energy, feeling content and confident in our body. What we eat and our lifestyles have a huge impact on our energy levels, our weight, our confidence and almost every aspect of our health and wellbeing. Yet, in most cases, what we eat and our lifestyle habits are not supporting us.

In 2008 we put a wholefood plant-based diet (more on this on page 10) to the test in our café above our veg shop in Ireland. We put 20 people on the diet for 4 weeks on what became the Happy Heart course. We didn't know if it would work, but we knew the research so far supported it. The results absolutely astounded us: all 20 reported having more energy, feeling lighter, and across the group there was an average drop in cholesterol of 20%, blood pressure was reduced to healthy levels, and there were many other positive side-effects.

After some media coverage of the results, we ended up making friends with doctors and brought them on board to develop even more medically-backed courses, centred around the power of a wholefood plant-based diet. We partnered with consultant gastroenterologist Dr Alan Desmond and NHS dietitian Rosie Martin, and together we created the Happy Gut course – a 6-week course to help improve people's digestive and gut health. Thousands of people have gone through this course and 98% would recommend it to a friend.

Since then we have created the Happy Skin course, in collaboration with Dr Gemma Newman and Jennifer Rock, aka The Skin Nerd, and also the Happy Shape Club, with Dr Sue Kenneally, NHS dietitian Rosie Martin, PT Zanna Van Dijk and yoga teacher Cliodhna Drury. To date we have had more than 35,000 people go through all of our courses from every corner of the world!

Although all our courses have a different focus, we have found that, because every part of our body is linked, when you start to heal one part of your body it will have a positive effect on the other parts too. If you have high cholesterol and follow our Happy Heart course, your cholesterol levels will most likely drop, and as your blood flow improves so too will your skin, as it gets more oxygen and nutrients. When you follow our Happy Gut course, your microbiome will start to consist of healthier 'gut bugs', and a healthier microbiome will mean that your taste buds change so that you crave healthier foods and it is a lot easier to maintain a Happy Shape and potentially lose excess weight. Once you start to make healthier food choices, you are more likely to get your 10,000 steps in a day, and once you are doing more walking you are more likely to meet others and connect; this will positively affect your sleep and your mental health is likely to improve too. One simple change starts a positive domino effect on your life!

The Happy Health Plan is not a diet. It's not a quick fix. It's not even a weight-loss plan (even though it can be very effective at this) – it is designed to change your life and your whole body health for good.

Based on everything we've learnt across our courses, the Happy Health Plan helps improve your heart health, your gut health, your skin, and it will help you reach your Happy Shape, along with lots of other positive benefits.

This book is the culmination of more than 10 years' experience of supporting tens of thousands of participants from all over the world as they positively change and transform their health with the power of a wholefood plant-based diet. Now it's your turn!

HOW TO USE THIS BOOK

If you want to focus on a particular area of your health, we've brought in the experts on our courses to give specific advice on:

- **Happy Heart:** improve your cardiovascular health and eat to reverse/avoid heart disease and high cholesterol.
- **Happy Skin:** improve the appearance of your skin and tackle common skin complaints and the effects of ageing.
- **Happy Shape:** lose weight and feel more confident in your body while also eating as much as you like of our plant-based recipes and following our really simple exercise tips.
- **Happy Gut:** aid your digestive system and tackle common complaints such as IBS, bloating and other tummy issues with our low-FODMAP, high-fibre recipes and our 6-week gut health programme.

Each section has expert advice, specific tips and carefully planned meal plans and shopping lists. You can either pick and mix across the sections or follow the plan to the letter, but either way we guarantee that you will start feeling better, have more energy and fall in love with plant-based foods. All we ask is that you do your best, choose progress over perfection and take it one step at a time.

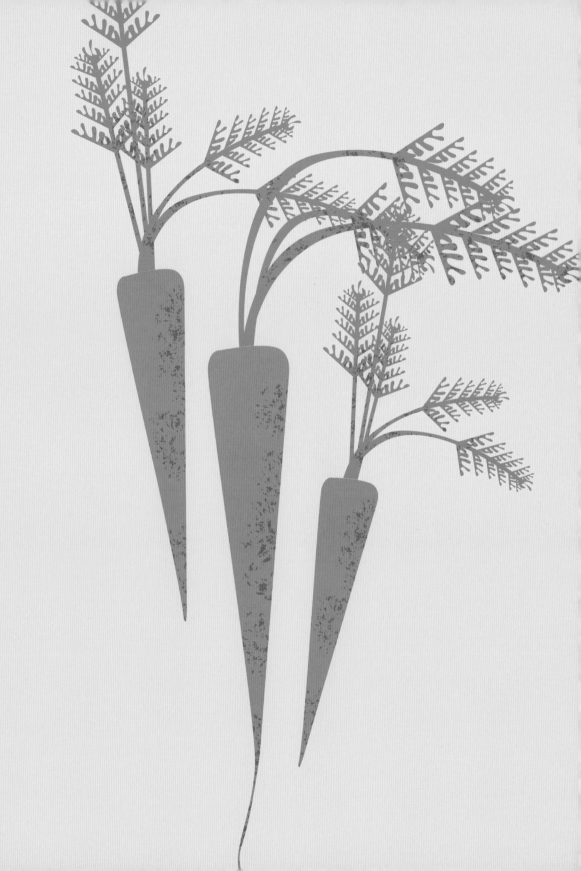

Chapter 1

Wholefood Plant-based Diet

Wholefood plant-based food is central to everything we do at The Happy Pear. Do you want to know the principles that have helped tens of thousands of people dramatically improve their health? Want to learn more about calcium and iron and why fibre is so important on our plans? It all awaits you in this chapter.

The food

The words 'wholefood plant-based diet' may be confusing, but basically 'wholefood' means eating foods as you would find them in nature rather than eating processed foods from a factory – and in case you were wondering, 'plant-based' is not referring to daffodils or roses but a diet made up of:

- Fruits
- Vegetables
- Beans (kidney beans, butter beans, black beans, etc.)
- Legumes (lentils, chickpeas, split peas, etc.)
- Wholegrains ('brown' carbs rather than 'white' carbs, or whole carbs as opposed to refined carbs)
- Nuts (raw nuts – not the roasted and salted type or the flavoured candied type nuts)
- Seeds (raw seeds such as sunflower, pumpkin, sesame, chia, flax, etc.)

In this book we explain how these incredible wholefoods provide all the nourishment our bodies need to thrive, including protein, which people often think is lacking in a plant-based diet. In fact, a diet made up of these delicious food groups is now what many professional athletes swear by. Our advice, meal plans and recipes in this book will give you the building blocks to embrace the power of plants and inspire you to give a wholefood plant-based diet a try for the benefit of your own health and wellbeing.

VEGAN DIET VS PLANT-BASED

The terms 'vegan' and 'plant-based' or 'wholefood plant-based' can often be mistaken for meaning the same thing, but this is not necessarily true.

A vegan diet is one that does not include any animal products or animal by-products, but that does not necessarily mean it is a healthy diet. You could live off chips, vegan biscuits, dark chocolate and cola and still be considered a vegan, but this is not any healthier than the standard Western diet.

A wholefood plant-based diet also does not contain any animal products but it is one that centres on unrefined and unprocessed wholefoods, and is made up of fruits, vegetables, wholegrains, legumes, nuts and seeds.

THREE TYPES OF FOOD

There are all sorts of different ways to look at food, but the way we find easiest to help us understand what foods are healthiest is to break them into the following three categories:

1. Whole plant-based foods
2. Refined foods
3. Animal-based foods (includes dairy and eggs)

Currently the average diet in the UK and Ireland in terms of calories consumed consists of something like:

5–10% Whole plant-based foods

50–55% Refined foods

40% Animal-based foods

The idea behind our Happy Health Plan is to move to a diet that is based on ideally 100% whole plant-based foods, or as close to it as you can get. Thinking of foods in terms of these three food groups takes a little bit of practice, but once you get your head around it, it becomes very easy to understand what foods are healthiest and what foods to avoid. Our recipes provide the perfect springboard into adopting this new way of eating and will help you to learn the ingredients and combinations that you enjoy the most.

Our plant-based principles

We have seen tens of thousands of people transform their lives by following these principles. They will have a hugely positive impact on your health and wellbeing – it's just a matter of giving them a shot. The list might seem like a lot, but just about everyone who finishes one of our courses says that it was a lot easier than they had initially thought and that the benefits far outweigh the effort. We know that everyone is starting from different experiences, so you don't need to do this all at once. Take it one step at a time and progress gradually.

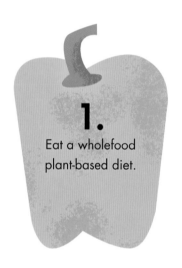

1.

Eat a wholefood plant-based diet.

2.

Eat as much as you like, no calorie-counting, no portion control, provided you are sticking to these 10 food principles.

55   205
183

3.

Use only wholegrain products.

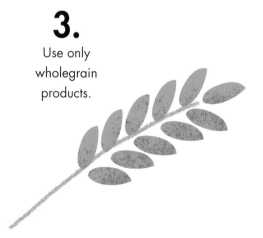

4.

Ensure that any packaged wholefoods that you eat have a fat content below 10%.

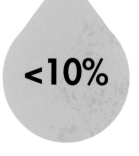

<10%

5.
Avoid refined or processed foods.

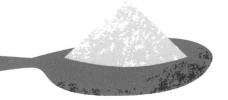

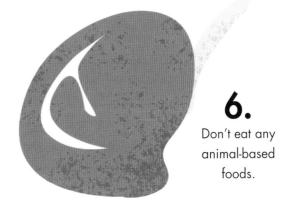

6.
Don't eat any animal-based foods.

7.
Avoid dairy products.

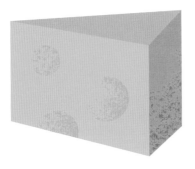

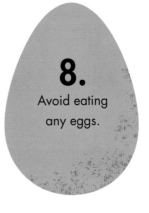

8.
Avoid eating any eggs.

9.
Avoid using any oil. That includes all oils: olive, sunflower, avocado, flax oil.

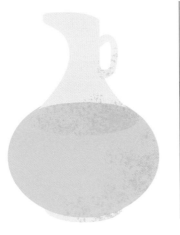

10.
Eat nuts, seeds and avocados sparingly.

Wholefood Plant-based Diet

Take a deep breath: we know this most likely comes across as very extreme, but let's break these down and explain why and how it works.

1. **Eat a wholefood plant-based diet**

   This is a diet based around 100% whole plant-based foods (or as close to it as you can get), as you would find them in nature – fruit, veg, beans, legumes, wholegrains, nuts and seeds.

2. **Eat as much as you like, no calorie-counting, no portion control, provided you are sticking to these 10 food principles***

   We know you think this can't be true, that no 'diet' lets you eat as much as you want, there must be a hook. Rest assured, there is no hook. It's because our food is:

   - Low energy density – our plans are made of food that is naturally low in calories while filling you up.
   - High in fibre – fills you up and takes longer to eat, and as a result your body registers that you are filling up quicker and reduces your hunger.
   - High in water – water in food has no calories but fills you up.

   * With the exception of our Happy Gut meal plan (page 118), as this is a controlled FODMAP approach and is very specific to rebuilding a healthy gut.

3. **Use only wholegrain products**

   Wholegrain products are the 'brown' carbs – brown rice, wholemeal pasta, wholemeal couscous, wholemeal noodles, 100% wholemeal bread. At least 80% of the carbohydrates we eat in the UK and Ireland are 'white' carbs, consisting of white pasta, white rice, white bread, pizza bases, doughnuts, etc. On our plans we want to replace these 'white carbs' that are low in fibre and missing much of their real nutrition with 100% brown carbs (see page 22 for more on this).

   Wholegrain products are:

   - High in fibre.
   - Low in calories.
   - Great sources of sustained energy – white carbs lead to energy spikes, brown carbs lead to more sustained energy.
   - Packed with nutrients – vitamins, minerals, antioxidants and phytonutrients.

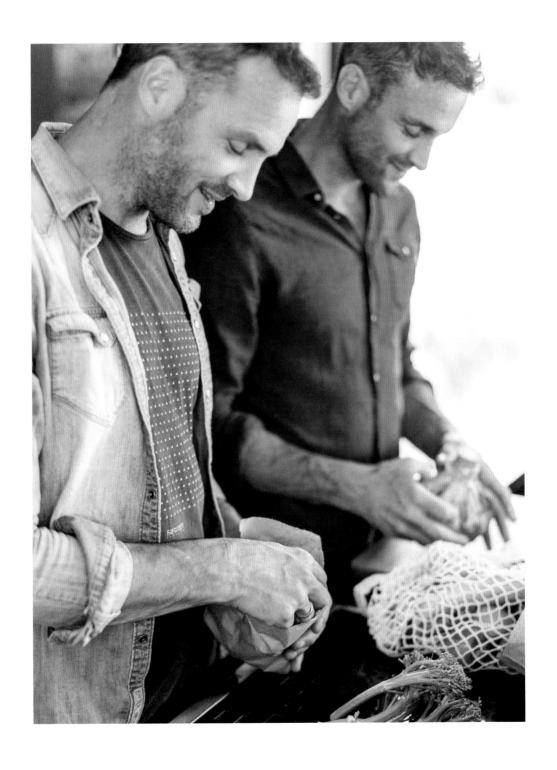

4. Ensure that any packaged wholefoods that you eat have a fat content below 10%

This ensures that the packaged foods you eat are still low energy density foods. To find out the % fat content of a product, simply turn to the back of the product's packet and look at the nutritional information. Fat will be listed in weight per the size of the product and per 100g. Simply look at the fat content per 100g and this will give you the percentage fat. For example, if I look at our organic red lentils below, the fat content per 100g is 1.3g, so the fat content for this product is 1.3%. Even some of our Happy Pears products don't quite fit these criteria, so it's always worth checking.

ORGANIC RED LENTILS
Nutrition values per 100g
Energy 213kcal/1325kJ
Fat 1.3g
Fat (of which saturates) 0.2g
Carbohydrates... 51g
Carbohydrates (of which sugars)......................... 2.4g
Protein 24g
Salt 0.04g
Fibre... 3.9g

5. Avoid refined or processed foods

Studies show that more than 50% of all calories consumed in the UK are from ultra-processed foods, and 45% in Ireland (estimated to be as high as 60% in the USA). These foods are convenient, affordable, highly profitable, strongly flavoured, aggressively marketed and on sale in shops and supermarkets virtually everywhere. The foods themselves will be familiar but the term ultra-processed may not be.

You might say that ultra-processed is just a sciency way to describe many of your normal, everyday foods and treats. It could be your morning bowl of cereal or your evening pot of flavoured yoghurt. It's pre-packaged savoury snacks and sweet baked goods. It's pizza on a Friday evening and vegan hotdogs. It's the chocolate cake you buy when you are being indulgent and the premium protein bar you eat at the gym to give you a lift. Consumed in isolation and moderation, each of these products may be OK – the problem is that the majority of the foods we are eating now are these ultra-processed foods.

Ultra-processed foods are packed with sugar, salt and fat and are considered 'empty calories', as they have little to no nutrition in them. They have little fibre in them to fill you up, making them easy to eat and hard to stop eating due to their high levels of fat, sugar and salt. This is really important and central to allowing you to eat as much as you want of the food on our plans (with the exception of Happy Gut).

6. Don't eat any animal-based foods

By animal-based foods we mean beef, lamb, chicken, turkey, ham, salami, sausages, bacon, and even fish, too. That is, red meat, white meat and fish – basically any food that had a face or a mother (sorry for being so crude!).

We exclude animal-based foods because:

- They are high in saturated and trans fats: both of these are considered the 'bad' fats that are linked to heart disease and diabetes.
- They contain no fibre: fibre is good for our gut, brain and weight.
- They contain cholesterol: excess cholesterol is associated with increased risk of heart disease. Our bodies produce all the cholesterol that we need; we do not need any extra from our diet.
- They are very low in antioxidants (the only antioxidants they contain are from the plants the animals consumed).
- They are low in vitamins and minerals compared to plant-based foods: see page 21.
- They often contain antibiotics and hormones: approximately 80% of antibiotics used globally are used in animal agriculture, along with growth hormones. Parts of these end up in meat and are believed to have a negative impact on your health, particularly your gut health.
- Animal-based foods contain only 2 of the 3 macronutrients: fat and protein. They are missing the number-one source of energy for your body: carbohydrates. In whole plant foods 20–80% of their calories come from carbs (most of these complex carbs), giving you a slow, sustained energy release.

7. Avoid dairy products

This means cheese, milk, butter and yoghurt made from animal milk. We know that living without butter and cheese is hard to imagine for some people, but we have found giving it up to be hugely beneficial to the health of people on our plan. We replace these with calcium-rich plant foods to keep our bones strong and cut out the foods that are associated with leaching calcium from our bones, such as high-protein

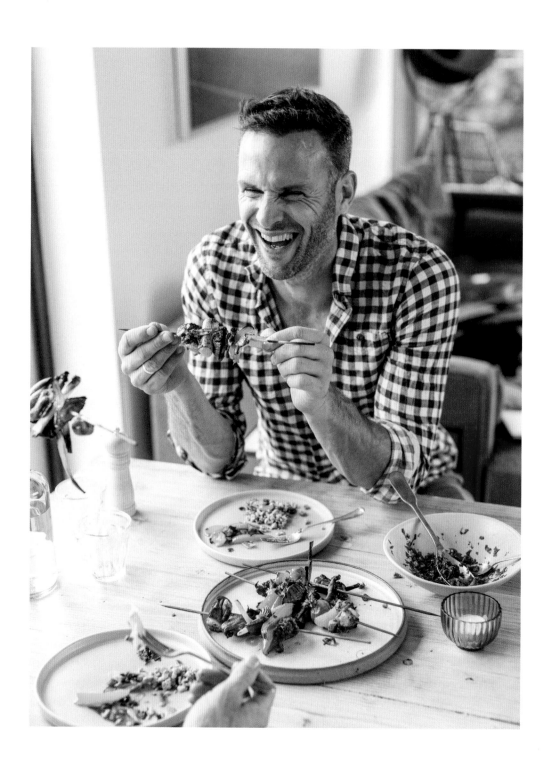

foods like meat and high-sodium foods such as processed foods (see page 26 for more on calcium). We have found cutting out dairy to be hugely effective in helping to lower cholesterol levels, stay in shape and improve lung function.

We exclude dairy products because:

- They are high in saturated fat and cholesterol, which are linked to heart disease.
- They contain no fibre.
- They contain little nutrition compared to whole plant foods: see page 21.

8. Avoid eating any eggs

We know lots of people love eggs, particularly at the weekend, but focus on the fact that our plans are for a few weeks only and that after that you can make your own mind up again. The reason eggs are excluded from our plan is that they are the most concentrated source of cholesterol in our diet. One large egg has about 200mg of dietary cholesterol in the yolk, the daily maximum limit of cholesterol in your diet being 300mg, or 200mg if you are at risk of heart disease. A recent study of nearly 30,000 people* showed that for each additional half egg eaten per day, there was a 6% higher risk of cardiovascular disease and an 8% higher risk of all-cause death. On page 21, see that 100 calories of broccoli is higher in every nutrient than eggs with the exception of cholesterol and fat, both of which you want to be lower.

* https://jamanetwork.com/journals/jama/fullarticle/2728487.

9. Avoid using any oil

This is the big one and so important for weight loss and for heart health. By oils we mean olive, sunflower, avocado, flax, etc. Cutting out oil is highly effective at lowering cholesterol, improving blood flow and skin, and also helping to lose weight, and you won't taste the difference – the food is just as delicious! We exclude oil because:

- It is high in empty calories – it has no fibre and very little nutrition and is the most calorie-dense food there is, at more than 8,000 calories per litre.
- It is 100% fat – no protein, carbohydrate and minimal nutrition other than fat.
- It contains no fibre, meaning that it won't fill you up but it is high in calories.
- It is high in saturated fat. Even olive oil is approximately 14% saturated fat; the daily recommended saturated fat intake is no more than 10%.
- It is a refined food that we extract from the wholefood, discarding the fibre and nearly all the vitamins and minerals, leaving us with nothing but the fat.

We are not against fat, but we recommend that you get your fat from wholefood sources such as small amounts of nuts, seeds, olives and avocados. Most people who start our courses think they could never cook without using oil, but page 25 shows how easy it is, and your taste buds adjust quickly to oil-free cooking. It is also much easier to wash your pots and pans after cooking.

10. Eat nuts, seeds and avocados sparingly

Here we mean raw nuts and seeds, not salted or roasted nuts/seeds, which are high in salt, less nutritious and hard to eat only a few of. Raw nuts and seeds are super-healthy and packed full of beneficial fats. However, we need only a very little of them. It's very easy to sit and eat a full bag while watching something on TV, or snacking between meals, but we need only a very little to get the real benefit from them, and going above this can cause inflammation (which is at the root of many diseases) and can have a negative effect on our gut, heart and weight.

We ask you to limit your intake of nuts to 30g a day, which is about:

- 20 almonds
- 10 walnuts
- 10 Brazil nuts
- 15 pecan nuts

The healthiest of all nuts (the highest in omega-3 – see page 31 – and the lowest in saturated fat) are walnuts. In terms of nut butters and tahini we ask you to limit them to a teaspoon a day, but it might just be easier to cut them out for the 4–6 weeks of the plan – they are so tasty that it is very difficult to stop at a teaspoon. We do include a little tahini and nut butter in some recipes, but in small quantities.

Like seeds and nuts, avocados are super-healthy for you. However, to optimize your heart health and to maintain a healthy weight, we encourage you to limit your avocado intake to a max of half an avocado every second day (if you keep the half with the stone in it in the fridge, it lasts well – or you can just share it). An avocado is about 300 calories, so they are higher in calories than most whole plant foods, with 20% coming from fat, although nearly all of this is the healthy type of fat.

Nutrient contents of 100 calories of broccoli, grilled sirloin steak, cheddar cheese and boiled eggs

	Broccoli	Grilled sirloin steak	Cheddar cheese	Boiled eggs
Calories	100	100	100	100
Protein	11.8g	15.4g	6.1g	9.9g
Fat	1.4g	4.2g	8.4g	6.7g
Calcium	126mg	3.2mg	177mg	38.5mg
Iron	2.2mg	1.2mg	0.07mg	1.4mg
Magnesium	60mg	14.3mg	7mg	9.8mg
Potassium	1,071mg	212mg	18mg	99mg
Fibre	10.9g	0g	0g	0g
Folate	207ug	9ug	7.4ug	21ug
Zinc	1.7mg	2.8mg	0.98mg	0.91g
Vitamin C	172mg	0mg	0mg	0mg
Vitamin A	175ug	0ug	93ug	84ug
Vitamin E	5.3mg	0.03mg	0.12mg	1.1mg
Cholesterol	0mg	37.6mg	23.3mg	252mg

Nutrition

It's important to know what these whole plant-based foods are made up of and what's so great about them, so here we've broken them down into their key components. We'll start by breaking down the three macronutrients (macros) within food – protein, carbohydrates and fats. These are the nutrients that the body uses in relatively large amounts and needs daily, whereas micronutrients, such as vitamins and minerals, are required in smaller amounts.

PROTEIN

Protein is primarily used by our bodies for growth and repair, and consists of 20 different amino acids, 11 of which can be made naturally by our bodies. The remaining 9 – which are called essential amino acids – must be ingested from our food. Our incredible bodies can mix and match different essential amino acids from the variety of foods we eat to make complete proteins. Great job, human body!

We live in a protein-obsessed society nowadays, where many people are eating protein to lose weight and just as many people are eating protein to gain weight. The vast majority of people think protein will give them energy, but the reality is that energy comes from carbohydrates and fat, not protein. In the West we can't seem to get enough protein, yet have you ever heard of anyone being diagnosed with a protein deficiency? Neither have we. Unless you are not eating enough calories or are simply existing on a diet consisting of refined and processed foods, it is very hard not to get enough protein.

If we were given €1 for every time someone asked us where we get our protein from (as we haven't eaten meat or any animal foods since 2001), we would be very wealthy men by now.

We can get all the protein we need from whole plant foods – even foods like lettuce and watermelon have protein in them. Most of the largest animals in the world – the elephant, rhino and gorilla – are plant-eating herbivores. These animals eat leaves and grasses and yet get more than adequate amounts of protein to build huge frames, much bigger than ours.

CARBS

It's very common to find people who are 'anti-carb' these days, but carbohydrates are not the problem. Carbohydrates are the main source of fuel for the body – they are good for you and vitally important. Fruits, veg, grains and beans are all packed with carbs; they form the fuel that our bodies function on for the central nervous system, energy for working muscles, and are also important for brain function, influencing mood and memory.

The problem is that since the 1980s in the West about 90% of carbohydrate intake is in the form of white flour, white pasta, white sugar and white rice. These refined carbs are often called 'empty calories', as they are stripped of their nutrients and are concentrated in calories. With white flour, for example, the whole grain is refined and stripped of its husk, germ and bran before being processed. You get a burst of energy after eating white carbs as well as a drop off or crash in energy when you have digested or absorbed these.

'Brown' carbs are higher in fibre, which means they are digested more slowly and give you a steadier, consistent release of energy, meaning no highs or lows in your energy levels and more consistent moods. They are much more nutritious, too. Whole carbohydrates include brown rice, brown pasta, wholemeal couscous, wholegrain bread, beans, vegetables and fruit. These carbs lead to sustained energy levels, better gut health and digestion, and even protect you from illness. Brown carbs also help you to lose weight or maintain a healthy weight as they are high in fibre, so they fill you up and give you a more consistent energy release with much fewer low points where you might have been prone to eating junk food. When you are in the supermarket and you are unsure whether a carb is white or brown, look out for 'whole' in front of the name, otherwise it is most likely a refined 'white' carbohydrate.

Instead of banning all carbs from your diet, embrace whole carbs and your body will thank you for it.

FATS

Fats are essential to our wellbeing: they provide energy, keep us warm, insulate our organs, and help us to absorb certain nutrients, to name a few functions. We encourage you to get your fats from wholefood sources such as small amounts of avocado, nuts and seeds, rather than from refined oils.

The message around fat is confusing: there seems to be so much conflicting research about 'heart healthy' olive oil and the miracles of coconut oil. Let's take a look at the basics.

Oils are man-made and are created by stripping away the fibre and nearly all the nutrients, leaving behind 100% fat. Oils have more than 8,000 calories per litre, the most calorie- and energy-dense substance on the planet. See the chart on page 24, illustrating the nutrition of the wholefood source of fat versus the stripped-down oil.

Nutrient contents of 100g of avocado, sunflower seeds and olives and their refined oils

	Avocado	Avocado oil	Sunflower seeds	Sunflower oil	Olives	Olive oil
Calories	160	884	584	884	115	884
Protein	2g	0g	20g	0g	1g	0g
Total fat	14.7g	100g	51.5g	100g	15.3g	100g
Carbs	8.5g	0g	20g	0g	6.3g	0g
Fibre	6.7g	0g	8.6g	0g	3.2g	0g
Calcium	12mg	0mg	78mg	0mg	88mg	1mg
Iron	7.5mg	0mg	5.2mg	0mg	3.3mg	0.6mg
Vitamin C	10mg	0mg	1.4mg	0mg	0.9mg	0mg
Saturated fat	2.1g	11.6g	4.5g	9.7g	1.4g	13.8g
Monounsaturated fat	9.8g	70.6g	18.5g	83.6g	7.9g	73g
Polyunsaturated fat	1.8g	13.5g	23.1g	3.8g	0.9g	10.5g

Notice that avocados, sunflower seeds and even salty olives are packed with nutrition, containing lots of fibre, carbohydrates and even protein when compared to the oils.

We encourage including whole fats in your diet, in moderation. By whole fats we mean whole plant foods that are naturally high in fat, such as avocados, nuts, seeds and olives. These fats contain all the fibre and the vitamins and minerals that our bodies are used to breaking down and assimilating.

TIP

HOW TO COOK OIL-FREE:

1. **Make sure to get a decent non-stick pan.** If you only have old ones and the seal is broken, then we would highly recommend that you buy a new one. All non-stick pans will say they are non-stick on the label.

2. **Make sure your pan is super-hot!** An easy way of knowing if your pan is hot enough is by dropping some water on to it. If it sizzles and evaporates in seconds, then your pan is hot enough. The reason for this is that the main way of developing flavour without oil is by browning your veg. The high heat will enable this.

3. **Deglaze your pan.** This might sound technical but it's actually a simple technique. As you are cooking your veg, there will be some browning happening which sticks to the bottom of the pan (some caramelized bits stick to the bottom). This 'browning' is packed with flavour for your dish, so add a few tablespoons of water/veg stock to the pan and scrape it off, using a wooden spoon/silicone spatula, and incorporate it into your sauce or food.

4. **Bake your vegetables.** Put your veg on a baking tray with some baking parchment. Baking your veg draws moisture out and concentrates the sweetness and flavour. Season them with a little salt – this will help to draw moisture out of the veg when baking and prevent them sticking too much to the tray.

CALCIUM

Calcium is a mineral, like iron, magnesium and copper, and all of these are found in the soil, where they are absorbed into the roots of plants. Animals like cows and sheep get their calcium by consuming these calcium-rich plants. So even though we are all conditioned to believe that calcium comes from cows' milk and dairy products, the real source of calcium richness is the soil. A varied diet of fruit, veg and wholefoods (without dairy) has plenty of calcium to meet all our needs. The best sources of easily absorbable calcium are plant foods such as dark green leafy vegetables like rocket, kale and watercress. Seeds are also an excellent source, particularly sesame seeds.

Calcium, bone health and avoiding osteoporosis

Bones are like muscles, in that they will only absorb calcium when they are stressed, just as muscles absorb protein when they are stressed. There are four parts to having sufficient calcium levels:

1. **Eating foods that contain calcium**, such as kale, lentils, seeds and beans. A lot of plant-based milks are also fortified with calcium.
2. **Minimizing the things that draw calcium from your body**, such as meat, coffee, refined foods that are high in salt, and smoking.
3. **Doing weight-bearing activities** – the primary cause of osteoporosis is not simply a lack of calcium but also a lack of physical activity, namely weight-bearing activity (e.g. walking, running, yoga). Weight-bearing activity strains the bones, the osteoblasts in our bones call out for more calcium and the calcium is absorbed.
4. **Vitamin D is also needed to absorb calcium.** Vitamin D works together with certain hormones to help the body absorb and use calcium. Most comes from sunlight, not diet, so it is important to spend time outside, but it can also be supplemented – see page 30 for more on this.

Once you are eating sufficient calories, a wholefood, plant-based diet will provide all the calcium you need. If you are pregnant, breastfeeding or have coeliac disease you may need to consult your doctor and be tested to ensure you are getting adequate levels.

IRON

Iron is an essential mineral that is part of all our cells. It provides oxygen to muscles, supports metabolism, and is also necessary for growth and development, to name a few of its properties. It is often presumed that eating a plant-based diet means you are more likely to suffer from low iron levels. However, studies have shown that those on a whole-food plant-based diet are no more likely to suffer from iron deficiency than omnivores.

Iron is found naturally in many different sources, such as wholegrains, beans, dark leafy greens, dried fruits, nuts and seeds. So eating a wide and varied whole-food plant-based diet naturally provides plenty of iron while containing no heme iron, which is linked to MS and heart disease and is found in animal-based foods.

It is said that plant-based iron is more easily absorbed by the body when eaten alongside foods high in vitamin C, so snacking on seeds and nuts with fruit, or serving beans with a tomato-based sauce, are great ways to combine this!

FIBRE

Fibre is one of the most important nutrients there is, and one that is so often overlooked. You only get fibre in fruit, veg, beans, legumes, wholegrains, nuts and seeds. Animal foods, fish, dairy products, eggs, and refined and processed foods have no fibre.

90% of people in the UK and Ireland don't reach their RDA (recommended daily allowance) of fibre. The average person gets about 17g of fibre per day, with the minimum daily requirement being 30g.

We see fibre as a good indicator of the health of a food – higher-fibre foods are nearly always associated with healthier, more nutrient-rich foods that also happen to be lower in calories.

To give an evolutionary context, if you look at the human diet throughout history the lack of fibre in our diet is only a fairly recent problem. For perhaps 99% of our existence, the human gut was packed daily with fibre-rich foods, and it was crucial to *Homo sapiens'* diet for thousands of years as we evolved into the modern human. It has only been in the last 100 years that our fibre intake has dropped dramatically and been replaced with processed and refined foods, leading to the massive increase in obesity, gut and digestive-related issues like IBS, as well as many of the other modern-day diseases that plague us today.

A WHOLEFOOD PLANT-BASED DIET, BY DIETITIAN ROSIE MARTIN

We have all heard the message that the diet and lifestyle choices we make contribute to our health and wellbeing, but do we understand the full power of our daily habits?

As a dietitian, I have studied food and nutrition for a number of years, and during this time I have supported a wide range of very different people and conditions. These vary from new diagnoses of coeliac disease, to people fighting heart disease and cancer. Food choices are a common and crucial factor in all of them. Although many areas of nutrition are hotly debated, the consensus around consuming whole and plant-based foods has almost always remained consistent; when it comes to plant foods, such as fruits, vegetables, beans and pulses, more is always better.

Across the board, studies of dietary patterns based on whole plant foods have shown that they consistently reduce our risk of chronic disease. A wholefood plant-based diet will reduce your chance of having high blood pressure, raised cholesterol, type 2 diabetes, and will support you to manage a healthy body weight, which in turn will reduce your chance of heart disease and strokes. It will also reduce your chance of developing diseases of the gut such as bowel cancer. The latest research is now highlighting the impact of our dietary patterns on our mood, and results indicate that improving your diet can make you happier!

A plant-based diet, as described by Steve and Dave, contains highly desirable levels of fibre, water, vitamins and minerals, and is lower in saturated fats and added sugars than other dietary patterns. As with any diet out there, ensuring it is well planned is an important factor. Due to our changing farming and food systems, as well as the change in our lifestyles over the time of human evolution, some vitamins and minerals now require special attention. For example, vitamin B12 and vitamin D are required in every diet, and may need supplementation to ensure a regular supply (see page 30 for more on this).

The combination of theoretical science and its application to practical meal plans and delicious recipes in this book creates a unique and valuable resource which I have seen support thousands of participants in taking control of their own health and wellbeing. I hope that it shows you, in a very tangible way, that improved health, wellbeing and happiness are just a few meal choices away. :)

Rosie Martin is a registered dietitian working within the NHS, with a special interest in disease prevention and plant-based nutrition. Rosie helped develop the Happy Gut and Happy Shape courses with us.
Instagram: @plantdietitianrosie

SUPPLEMENTATION, BY DR ALAN DESMOND

Whether you're completely plant-based, flexitarian or omnivore, there are three key nutrients that you need to know about.

Vitamin B12 is produced by bacteria in the soil. Meat contains vitamin B12, because the animals have either ingested these bacteria while grazing or have themselves been given supplements. It is vital in maintaining healthy brain function, regulating the production of DNA and the formation of the red blood cells that carry oxygen around our bodies.

Because our fruits and vegetables are now cleaned of any soil prior to eating, they no longer come with a source of vitamin B12. We don't recommend eating soil, due to the risk of contracting diseases, but we do strongly recommend taking a vitamin B12 supplement.

One simple and affordable option is called Veg-1, available from www.vegansociety.com. It contains a daily dose of vitamin B12, enough for the majority of people. For a minority of people, higher doses are required. Vitamin B12 deficiency is common whatever your dietary choices, so if you are suffering from fatigue, or if you are a woman planning a pregnancy, please get your level checked.

Vitamin D3 appears in small amounts in certain foods, but our bodies have evolved to make their own supply. Active vitamin D is manufactured in our skin, but this process depends on exposure to strong sunlight. Deficiency has been linked to increased risk of heart disease, fractured bones, memory problems and high blood pressure.

Because our modern lives tend to keep us indoors, vitamin D deficiency is incredibly common, whether we are omnivore, vegetarian or vegan. The UK Scientific Advisory Committee on Nutrition recommends that everyone should take a vitamin D supplement during the winter months, or all year round if they work indoors.

While you can obtain small amounts of vitamin D from foods such as tofu and mushrooms, and from fortified plant-based milks, if you cannot guarantee 20 minutes of bright sunshine 365 days a year, we strongly recommend that you take 400 international units or 10 micrograms of vitamin D each day. A convenient way to take this is in the Veg-1 supplement. Higher doses of vitamin D can be harmful, so never take more than 2,000 international units daily without medical supervision.

Omega-3 fatty acids are one type of a group of healthy oils, also known as polyunsaturated fatty acids. There are two types of omega-3, short-chain and long-chain. Both are important to help maintain your long-term brain and heart health.

You can get enough short-chain omega-3 by eating a tablespoon of chia seeds, flax seeds or walnuts each day. But long-chain omega-3s are a bit trickier. One great source of these is algae. Because fish eat a lot of algae, eating oily fish or taking a fish-oil supplement is one option. However, on a healthy plant-based diet, we prefer to bypass the middle-fish, by taking 250mg of a plant-based omega-3 supplement daily. There are lots of brands available; most are made by extracting omega-3-rich oil directly from algae. The science does not clearly show that long-chain omega-3 supplementation is mandatory when following a 100% plant-based diet, but many doctors and dietitians advise it.

Dr Alan Desmond, MB, BCh, BMedSc, MRCPI, FRCP, is a consultant gastroenterologist and author of The Plant-Based Diet Revolution.
Instagram: @dr.alandesmond

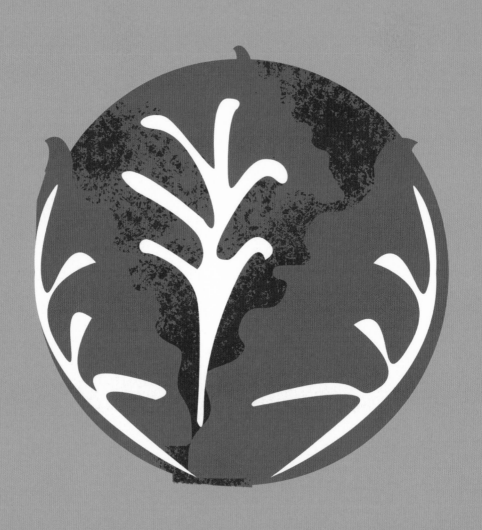

Chapter 2

Lifestyle

As human beings our life and work revolve around food, but they are not the only factors in a healthy lifestyle. How much we move, the quality of our sleep, our social connections and how we deal with stress all have a part to play in being fit and healthy.

Movement

In the afternoon when you feel tired and experience a slump, what do you turn to for more energy to give you a boost? Most of us turn to chocolate, sweet snacks, energy drinks, coffee or some form of food or drink that we think will give us a lift. Yet our primary fuel source is not food or even water but oxygen, which we get through movement. Once you move, oxygen is pumped around your body, bringing with it nutrients and charging up your mitochondria, your body's energy powerhouses. While it may sound like a contradiction, if you are looking to have more energy and beat the afternoon slump, there is no better way than to get moving!

Some of the benefits of regular movement:

- It releases endorphins that make you feel good.
- It increases energy.
- It enhances sleep.
- It lowers chances of obesity and chronic disease.
- It tends to encourage you to be more social.

On average in the UK, adults spend a whopping 9½ hours a day sitting (slightly less in Ireland), which actually equates to more time sitting than sleeping in any given day. Not surprisingly, in Western countries 36% of all people are sedentary (i.e. do not move enough, which is considered as walking less than 5,500 steps per day). This is more than double the percentage in developing countries, and interestingly enough women tend to be more sedentary than men, with 40% of women in the UK not moving enough and 32% of men.*

In a sense, sitting is the new smoking of our time. It is at the root of so many ailments and diseases. You probably inherently know that sitting is poor for your health, but to drill a little deeper, excessive sitting negatively affects your immune system, your energy levels, your mental health, as well as your muscle mass.

* *Lancet*, https://www.who.int/ncds/prevention/physical-activity/Worldwide-trends-physical-inactivity-press-release.pdf?ua=1.

MOVEMENT MAKES YOU HAPPIER

How many times a day do you think young kids smile? The answer is about 400 times a day on average, and young kids move around a huge amount – they are not very good at sitting still. Adults, on the other hand, tend to be experts at sitting still. The average adult

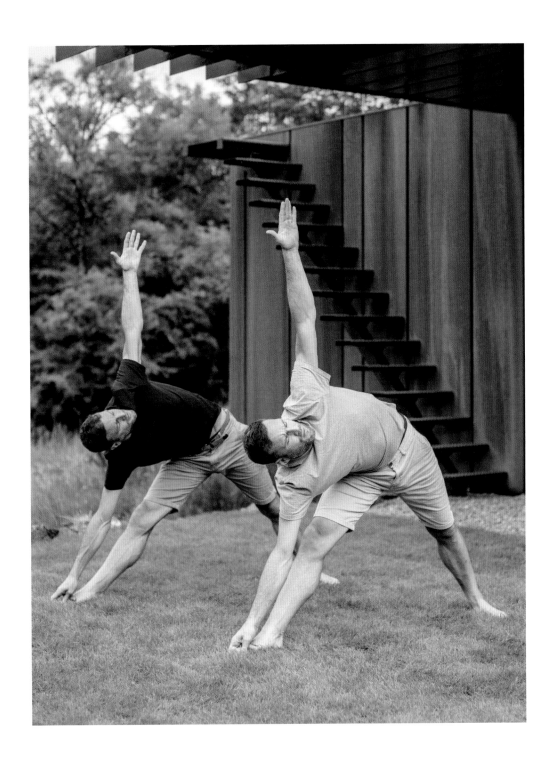

smiles only 20–30 times a day, and a more upbeat adult smiles 40–50 times. Movement is so important to our mental health – it releases endorphins and hormones in our brain that make us feel good, more optimistic, as well as giving us more oxygen, which in turn leads to more energy.

BEING ACTIVE THROUGHOUT THE DAY IS WHAT COUNTS

Research shows that consistent movement throughout the day is more effective in terms of energy levels and avoiding disease, even when compared to active people who sit most of the day but do vigorous exercise an hour a day. Researchers found that consistent movement was better for physical condition, mental alertness, better mental health and stress reduction than short bursts of vigorous physical activity. Consistent movement is key.

Target 10,000 daily steps

Getting into the habit of actually checking and monitoring your daily steps is a basic tool that is hugely effective: the goal is to get to 10,000 steps a day, which roughly equates to about 5 miles. As previously mentioned, people who walk less than 5,500 steps a day are considered sedentary and in the UK the average number of steps is just 5,836 (in Ireland studies suggest it is more like 8,000 steps a day). The very simple action of measuring your steps actually improves your numbers. Your mobile phone can most likely count your steps, and if you prefer a more visible accurate reminder, there are any number of wearable health gadgets that will do it.

Top tips for getting your 10k steps in

- Little and often: a few regular steps are better than one big walk. It's better to constantly move through the day, than be sedentary the majority of the time.
- Reclaim your lunch break: use your lunchtime to get outdoors into the fresh air and walk, even just for 10 minutes.
- Walk and talk: take any meetings or catch up with friends outside, and walk and chat.
- Mobile phones: put in your headphones and make your phone calls while you walk.
- Take the stairs: choose the stairs over the lift or escalator.

- Your stop: if you use public transport, get off the bus or train one stop early and walk the rest of the way.
- Priority parking: park furthest away from the supermarket door and walk the rest of the way.
- Get a dog: they make the world's best walking coaches!

Advice for starting exercising
- Schedule your walks/workouts in your diary, just like you would do with a work meeting or a coffee with a friend.
- It can often help to do a walk/workout in the morning, before the day begins and pulls you off course.
- Small amounts are best to begin with – if you are not used to being active, start with even 10-minute walking intervals throughout the day and gradually build up to 30–40 minutes at a time.
- Find an activity that you enjoy – it can be anything from walking to gardening – the more you enjoy something the more likely you are to do it.
- Ask a friend or family member to join in! Why not get your partner or housemate to do some form of movement/workout with you!
- Remember that all types of movement count: taking the stairs, housework and gardening are all great ways to fit exercise into the day. There are so many different types of exercise that it's a good idea to try out various activities and see what you enjoy. From hill-walking to surfing, from yoga to gardening, there is something out there for everyone! So, what are you waiting for? Lace up your trainers, get out and get moving!

MINDFULNESS

We haven't got the space to delve into the meditation or mindfulness side of health in this book, unfortunately, but it is important to us. We both meditate most mornings, as it helps activate that really important inner world and helps us to be less reactive and more mindful. We encourage you to develop this side of your health too, as it is so rewarding and will further amplify the positive impact of the Happy Health Plan.

Sleep

Sleep is one of the foundations of health and wellbeing, enhancing the function of just about every organ in the body and every process in the brain. We both get up early in the morning, we always have done, usually rising just after 5. Many people make the assumption that we function on not very much sleep, and are usually quite surprised when we tell them that we get into bed around 9 every night. According to research, around 40% of people are like us 'early birds', and evening-type 'owls' account for about 30%, preferring to go to bed late and wake up late. The remaining 30% are somewhere in between.

As a society, we are in a sleep crisis. More than 60% of us are not getting our 7–8 hours of sleep a night as recommended by the World Health Organization. A recent study revealed that in 1942, less than 8% of the population was trying to survive on 6 hours or less sleep a night, but by 2017 that proportion was up to almost 1 in 2 people. It is an epidemic and is having serious ramifications on all aspects of our lives.

Without sleep, there is low energy and disease. With sleep, there is vitality and health. More than 20 large-scale studies report the same clear relationship: the shorter your sleep, the shorter your life.

In the short term, poor sleep can have an impact on your mood, your productivity, your food choices and your interactions. In the long term, it's been linked to serious medical issues like heart disease, stress, poor memory function, reduced ability to fight infection, weight gain, increased risk of type 2 diabetes and depression.

Each of us will benefit greatly from prioritizing sleep. It's one of the cheapest health 'superfoods' there is!

TIP

10 TIPS TO SET YOURSELF UP FOR BETTER SLEEP:

1. **Regularity.** Be consistent with the time that you go to bed and the time you wake.
2. **Routine.** Form a bedtime routine. This might be reading a book or taking a bath to actively try to wind down.
3. **Prioritize your sleep.** Don't cut sleep for the sake of entertainment or socializing, as this will spill out into every area of your life.
4. **No screens an hour before bed.** Reducing screen time before sleep greatly aids in giving your brain less stimulation and the space it needs to start to unwind.
5. **Keep your phone out of the bedroom while you sleep.** Buy an old-school alarm clock and leave your phone in another room so that you are not tempted to look at it.
6. **Lower the temperature.** Open the window in your bedroom to lower the temperature before you hit the sheets – a lower-temperature bedroom helps your body to cool down and initiate sleep.
7. **Dim the lights.** Try to minimize bright artificial light exposure before going to bed. Actively dim the lights right down.
8. **Try again.** If you can't sleep for more than 20 minutes, get out of bed and do something quiet and relaxing until the urge to sleep returns.
9. **Avoid caffeine after 1 p.m. and avoid going to bed tipsy.** Alcohol is a sedative and sedation is not sleep. It also blocks your REM dream sleep, an important part of the sleep cycle.
10. **Keep it dark.** Don't turn on the light if you go to the toilet during the night, as it will only interrupt your body's sleep cycle.

Community

The most basic physiological human need is for connection. Underneath all our materialistic desires is the need to feel connected, to belong, to feel a part of something. As a species we evolved on the plains of Africa, and we didn't survive through being the biggest, fastest or strongest – the reason we survived was because we are very good at working together, at being part of a tribe. Community, connection and belonging are built into our DNA; we are not made for isolation.

CURRENT SITUATION

In January 2018, the UK government appointed its first minister for loneliness, following on from results of a study in 2017 which showed that 9 million people in the UK often or always feel lonely: that is a huge 14% of the population. A recent study found loneliness to be 'associated with a reduction in lifespan similar to that caused by smoking 15 cigarettes a day'. Loneliness is becoming an epidemic.

Loneliness is usually associated more with older people suffering from social isolation, but the UK Office for National Statistics (ONS) found that 16–24-year-olds reported feeling more lonely than pensioners between the ages of 65 and 74. Technology, like mobile phones, is seen as a source of isolation for many young people, with many studies linking an over-attachment to mobile phones to feelings of anxiety and loneliness, but at the same time it can be a solution for older generations, keeping them connected to their families.

Steve and I have five kids, not together, but between us. When we take our young kids to the playground we've seen them run straight up to another kid and say, 'Hi, can I be your friend?' and they have made a friend, it's that simple! As adults, it tends to be a bit more complex, with many of us using different strategies to stand out from the crowd and show our value, such as gaining lots of money or having a strong body, but underneath all our strategies to gain connection, influence or status is the need to belong. We like to think that as adults we are all walking around with invisible signs that say, 'I am worthy, please love me and be my friend'; the most basic need is for connection, yet most of us pretend we don't want it or need it.

We believe that the power of the collective, that community, is the bedrock of health and happiness and that we all need the support and encouragement of others in order to evolve and grow. Ultimately that is why we set up The Happy Pear in 2004, with the aim of creating a community of people who could help to make the world a healthier, happier place!

Support from those around you is so important if you want to make any positive lifestyle changes; we all know what we need to do in terms of improving our health, but what can sometimes hold us back from succeeding is the lack of a support network around us.

FINDING OUR TRIBE

When we went travelling in 2001, back in the days before The Happy Pear, we left Ireland as rugby-playing, beer-drinking, burger-loving, alpha-male-type characters. Two years later, we came back a pair of vegans, who did not drink alcohol and who were into yoga, the power of community, and making the world a happier, healthier place! Our old friends didn't know what to think of us, they couldn't relate to us, so we had to find a new tribe and build a community of people who were into the same type of lifestyle that we were into and who would support us – and so we began The Happy Pear! We inherently knew that if we didn't cultivate another community of people that were into our new lifestyle we wouldn't be able to sustain it in the long run.

The Happy Pear stood for everything we were about and it attracted people who were into the same lifestyle that we were into. From it, a wonderful community of positive people started to form and enrich our lives.

4 TIPS TO BUILD COMMUNITY

1. **Awareness** – It all starts with being aware that as humans, we are social creatures and have a need to be part of a community to thrive.
2. **Start saying hello to people in your neighbourhood** – This might sound incredibly simplistic, but by simply acknowledging and greeting your neighbours, community will follow.
3. **Be proactive** – Join a club/group with the focus on making connections; in today's society, where loneliness is so common, you will probably need to be proactive rather than waiting for connections to randomly happen. As adults, we typically need a reason to hang out, whether it be exercise, travel, going for coffee, etc.
4. **Be real, show vulnerability** – Connection starts with yourself, connecting with who you are. Being authentic and vulnerable and honest about cultivating connections and community will only help.

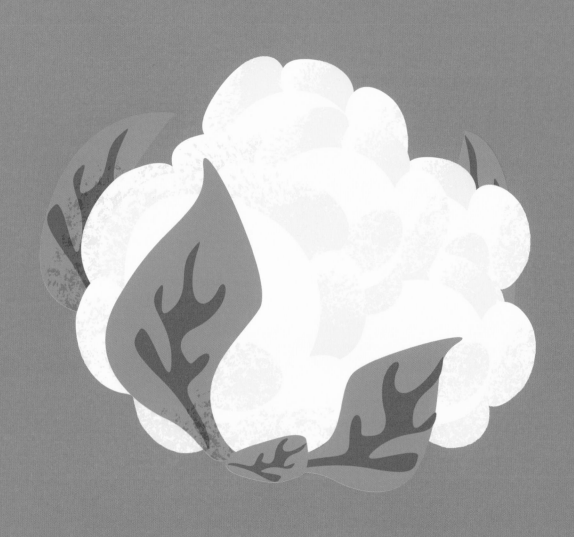

Chapter 3

Happy Heart

We started running our Happy Heart course upstairs in our café back in 2008. We had been eating a wholefood plant-based diet for about 7 years and were feeling the benefits, so we wanted to put it to the test.

Starting our Happy Heart plan

We had read about Dr Dean Ornish's lifestyle heart trial, where he showed in clinical trials that in 83% of his cases all the indicators for heart disease were not just halted but were actually reversed by eating a wholefood plant-based diet over the year of his study. Today we have had more than 20,000 people go through our Happy Heart course in more than 73 countries, with results in 4 weeks that often leave people amazed. Below we outline how to optimize your heart health for more energy, lower cholesterol levels, lower blood pressure and even weight loss.

We recommend that prior to starting your 4-week Happy Heart culinary adventure you get starting measurements so that you can compare before and after. We use cholesterol levels, blood pressure and weight, and you can use blood sugar levels too. You can get these done at your local doctor's surgery, though conditions may vary in different areas. Turn to page 106 for a sample meal plan and shopping list, or pick and mix from the heart-healthy recipes with a next to them.

"

For the best part of 20 years (half my life!) I've been trying to reduce my cholesterol. I have a family history of heart disease, heart bypasses and all sorts of heart-related health adventures. I've tried lots of different ways to control my cholesterol, from exercise (I've competed in marathons and triathlons), to diet (from drinking plant sterol yoghurts to going pescatarian), but have failed to find anything that will have much of a lasting impact.

With the arrival of my daughter into my life, the need to do something to avoid the threat of a heart attack became more urgent. Knowing how anxious I was about this, my siblings very generously bought me the Happy Heart course as a birthday gift.

It was life-changing. The plan was easy to stick to. The recipes are tasty, and practical, and the results speak for themselves. My cholesterol levels almost halved and I lost more than 4 kilos in weight. I felt physically and metaphorically lighter – like the bogeyman of heart disease had been banished. It was hugely emotional.

Since then, I've continued to lose weight and have convinced other family members to follow in some of my footsteps, and their results have been equally exciting. I owe the Happy Pear lads a huge debt of gratitude for nothing less than adding what I hope will be another number of happy and healthy years to my life.

– Patrick

By heart health we mean having arteries with no plaque blockages, where blood flows freely to and from our heart to all parts of our body. Oxygen, our primary fuel source, and nutrients are passed around our body to every cell via our blood supply, so having a healthy blood flow and cardiovascular health is foundational to good overall health.

In terms of heart disease the current situation is not pretty at all. It is the number-one killer in the world, with nearly 1 in 2 dying from CVD (cardiovascular disease) in Europe, and globally nearly 1 in 3. It accounts for nearly 170,000 deaths in the UK each year – that's an average of 465 people each day or one death every 3 minutes.

However, the good news is that in the vast majority of cases not only can heart disease be halted in its tracks, but many of the signs can actually be reversed. Even better news is that in nearly all cases, the power lies in your hands: we have shown through our Happy Heart course that lifestyle changes such as what you eat, the amount you move and how you deal with stress can have a massive impact on improving your heart and overall health and wellbeing.

As Dr Kim Williams (President of the American College of Cardiology 2015 and Chief of Cardiology at Rush University in Chicago) says: 'There are two types of cardiologists, vegans and those that haven't yet read the data.'

My relationship to food is completely different. I have always loved cooking for others but now I love cooking for me too. I'm more confident that this way of eating is right for me. I definitely had more consistent energy while doing the course.

– Ruth

An overview

The likely outcomes of 4 weeks on this Happy Heart plan are:

- **Lower cholesterol levels:** the average cholesterol reduction we see from participants is 20% in just 4 weeks.
- **Improved blood pressure:** we usually see high blood pressure drop in the 4 weeks.
- **Weight loss:** we encourage you to eat as much Happy Heart food as you like and you will still lose weight if you need to, no calorie-counting and no portion control.
- **More energy:** better blood flow equals more oxygen and nutrients to your cells, which equals more energy!
- **Regulate your blood sugars:** we have had many type 2 diabetics through the course and their blood sugar levels tend to regulate to normal healthy levels during the 4 weeks.
- **Better sleep:** participants very often report improved sleep.
- **Wellbeing:** a lightness and general improvement in overall wellbeing.

THE CHINA STUDY

In the famous China Study, researchers led by Dr T. Colin Campbell followed the mortality rates and their link to the diet of hundreds of thousands of rural Chinese people. In one rural Chinese province of more than half a million people who subsisted on a wholefood plant-based diet with very small amounts of animal-based foods, not a single death was blamed on heart disease over a period of 3 years. Taking the UK average, an area the size of Manchester, with a similar population of 500,000 people, would suffer over 1,000 deaths from CVD per year.

The twins, David and Stephen Flynn, chefs by profession, have developed a programme that is clearly the future of health and the practice of medicine. It is an extraordinary story whose time has come.

– Dr T. Colin Campbell, co-author of the international bestseller The China Study *and leading scientist on the effects of diet on disease.*

It was a shock to be told that I had had a heart attack in May of this year. I was admitted to hospital and had three stents fitted. My eldest daughter suggested to me that I join up to the Happy Heart course for one month. I was happy to have a chance to do something about my health. I lost 10kg during the course and my health is continuing to improve.

– Frank

OTHER FACTORS AFFECTING HEART DISEASE WHICH WE ARE NOT FOCUSING ON HERE

Heart disease is a very complex issue and there are many other contributing factors to heart health that the plan doesn't cover but which should definitely be looked into alongside the plan with your doctor if you have any heart-health issues.

- Smoking – we recommend quitting, as smoking is a leading factor in heart-related illnesses.
- Diabetes – for type 2 diabetics we have found our Happy Heart course very effective at improving and even regulating blood sugar levels.
- Inactivity – start striving towards getting your 10,000 steps a day (see page 36).
- Alcohol consumption – as with smoking, we also suggest that alcohol consumption should be reduced to the recommended weekly amount, as it can also be detrimental to good heart health.
- Stress – trying to reduce your stress levels is key. Consistent movement/ exercise and good sleep are two factors that help buffer against stress, but other practices such as yoga and meditation and any activities that bring you back to the present moment are beneficial.

I lost about 10lb during the course and I have more energy now. The focus of the course wasn't on eating less and being hungry, it was about cooking tasty food and being full. I definitely cook more, and when snacking, I choose healthier alternatives. I don't crave chocolate and biscuits like I did before. I won't be going back to my old diet. I will only be expanding my Happy Heart-friendly recipes and eating more veggies than ever before!

– Vicki

THE DEVON SOUTH-WEST PLANT-BASED CHALLENGE

In January 2020 we embarked on a study which we called the South-West Plant-Based Challenge. Dr Alan Desmond wanted to show the power of a plant-based diet to his fellow medical professionals. We enrolled 75 doctors, nurses, dietitians and other medical professionals and got them on a wholefood plant-based diet for 4 weeks. Almost every participant had been eating an omnivorous diet before starting the course, for an average of 49 years!

The findings after 4 weeks were as follows:

- Average total cholesterol drop was 20%. Only 35% of the group had normal cholesterol levels starting the challenge, and 4 weeks later 77% of the group had normal cholesterol levels.
- There was an average of 3.2kg weight loss across the participants, with the biggest weight loss in the group being 9.5kg.
- 37% of the group started the challenge overweight/obese, and after the 4 weeks only 27% were in the overweight/obese group.
- Those with the highest starting cholesterol and BMI reduced their 5-year risk of coronary vascular disease by at least a third.
- Blood pressure reduced from an average of 121/76 to 114/74, as effective as prescribing a first-line blood pressure medication.
- 74% of participants decided to make the switch to a plant-based diet permanently.
- 97% of participants thought they should offer a similar programme to their patients!

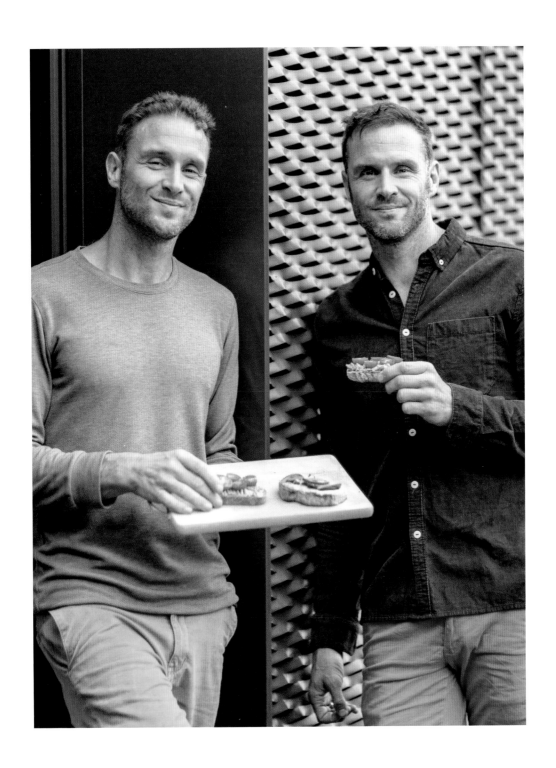

DR JOEL KAHN, MD, AMERICA'S HEALTHY HEART DOCTOR

As a Happy Heart doc, I am so excited about the Happy Heart. I adopted a wholefood, plant-only diet 43 years ago at age 18 and I have never eaten an animal-based food since. I maintained this even while graduating medical school number-one and completing training as an interventional cardiologist placing balloons and stents for heart attacks. Oddly, 3 weeks after I began my career, Dean Ornish, MD published the Lifestyle Heart Trial, demonstrating the reversibility of even long-established heart disease (using a plant-based diet, stress management, group support, and fitness). From then on, every one of the tens of thousands of patients I have cared for has been taught that a wholefood plant-based diet is a powerful therapy to prevent and reverse heart disease. In my preventive clinic, I use advanced carotid ultrasound scans and routinely confirm the reversal of narrowed arteries by educating patients on wholefood plant-based diets and lifestyle measures. Let me say it again, I see clogged arteries get younger and younger as a routine benefit of a wholefood plant-based diet. At age 61 I recently had both my carotid and heart arteries scanned and they are completely free of any plaque, even though my family history of cholesterol and heart disease is not favourable.

Why do wholefood plant-based diets without added oils provide so much protection for our arteries? We have about 80,000 kilometres of arteries in our bodies. Each segment is lined by a single layer of cells called the endothelium, which acts like a thin wallpaper in our arteries. The endothelium itself has another coating called the glycocalyx, which further protects our miraculous arteries. When we smoke, or eat fatty meats high in saturated fat, hormones, antibiotics, pesticides and newly discovered chemicals like neu5Gc, we damage the glycocalyx and the endothelium and we begin the downward spiral of developing high blood pressure, erectile dysfunction in men, and clogged arteries. On the other hand, when we eat whole fruits, vegetables, 100% wholegrains and legumes, we maximize our nutrient intake including vitamin C and we strengthen both the glycocalyx and the endothelial cells. Eating for your arteries, with lots of greens, red foods like apples, bell peppers, pomegranates and berries, and avoiding excess added sugar calories and oils, is the ticket to a happy ride through life with happy arteries.

Does a wholefood plant-based diet guarantee you will never have a heart attack? Sadly, there is no 100% warranty, but it is the only diet proven by decades of scientific studies to prevent and reverse the number-one killer in the Western world. In addition to your diet, get regular exercise, in nature if possible, aim for 7 hours of sleep, don't smoke, stay lean, and have strong social connections and a sense of purpose in life. Finally, know your numbers. Measure your blood pressure often and know your fasting blood sugar, cholesterol panel, lipoprotein(a) genetic cholesterol level, and perhaps your inflammation status by checking your hs-CRP. Together your life will be happy, your arteries will be happy, the planet will be happy, and the animals you did not eat will definitely be happy.

Joel Kahn, MD, FACC, is Clinical Professor, Wayne State University School of Medicine. A cardiologist since 1983, he is the author of The Whole Heart Solution *and the bestselling* America's Healthy Heart Doc. *We developed the Happy Heart course with Dr Kahn.*
Instagram: drjkahn
https://www.drjoelkahn.com/

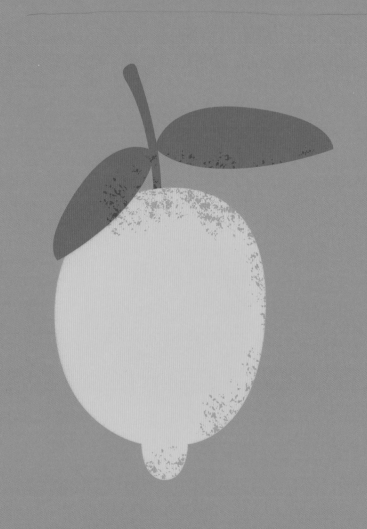

Chapter 4

Happy Skin

Your skin is like the fruit of a tree – the sweetness and deliciousness of the fruit depends on so many variables, such as the soil, the nutrients, the light levels and the rain it receives. Likewise your skin is a reflection of the health of your body, how you live your life, what you eat, how you sleep, your level of physical activity and how at ease you are. For sure, genetics has a role to play but, as with many modern illnesses, your lifestyle is the real decider.

Happy Skin pillars

- **Adopt a wholefood plant-based diet,** which is naturally packed with antioxidant, anti-inflammatory, fibre- and water-rich foods, to help your skin glow. Look for recipes with for inspiration.
- **Cut out refined and processed foods** that are low in water, high in added fat and sugar, which age and damage your skin through inflammation.
- **Eat antioxidant-rich foods** (lots of bright-coloured fruits and veggies) – these help reduce free radical damage to your skin.
- **Eat omega-3-rich plant foods** (walnuts, flax seeds, chia seeds, algae, seaweeds), which help keep your skin hydrated.

> **"**
>
> Before I did the Happy Skin course, I had struggled with breakouts on my skin for 2 years. I had visited the GP, had tried multiple antibiotics and nothing was working to clear it. After having no luck with any other skin treatments I thought I had nothing to lose, so I signed up.
>
> I found that planning the week's meals in advance and buying food for a specific recipe meant less food waste and saved me time. As I work 'unsociable hours', I mostly batch cook for work meals, and I found it great that a lot of the meals are freezer-friendly. The recipes were very simple to follow, quick to prepare, not complex to cook and, most importantly, tasted delicious.
>
> The focus of the course was on eating a wholefood plant-based diet as opposed to just eating vegan. The aim was all about eating as much fruit, vegetables and fibre as possible. I noticed there was no focus on restrictions; it was more what I could eat as opposed to what I couldn't. It wasn't just about the food, either; we were encouraged to monitor our general health and wellbeing. This was done by keeping a weekly diary of daily water intake, stress levels and exercise taken, to name just a few.
>
> I knew the cooking and the food wouldn't be an issue but I didn't expect to like the course as much as I did. Any time I was cooking at

home or having lunches in work I always got a lot of positive comments. The dramatic difference to my skin after 4 weeks was something I didn't expect. My skin is clearer and much brighter now.

This course has made a significant impact on my overall diet and I continue to eat a mostly wholefood plant-based diet. The Happy Pear have a great philosophy: eat good, wholesome plant-based food and feel great!

– Jane

The Happy Skin plan helped me to understand more about my skin type and how to look after it. Learning ways to get my skin looking more hydrated was brilliant, and my friends commented on how great my skin was looking too! The food not only helped my skin to look better – I had more energy too!

– Claire

EXPERT FOCUS

DR GEMMA NEWMAN, THE PLANT-POWERED DOCTOR

We can often get so caught up in how our skin looks, what blemishes, freckles or wrinkles it has, that it can be hard to appreciate all the other incredible things our skin does to keep us safe and healthy. It can be easy to forget that our skin isn't purely aesthetic and that it is, in fact, the largest organ of the body. The skin's job is to protect us: it keeps the good stuff in and the bad stuff out. It protects us from UV light. It helps to regulate our body temperature and prevents water loss, and it is responsible for the secretion of oils. The skin is also a hormonally active organ, the site of vitamin D production, and it contains immune system cells which help to protect us from infection. It is also a sensory organ, allowing us to enjoy the sensation of physical touch from our nearest and dearest. Now you can hopefully appreciate that there is so much more to the skin than what it looks like on the outside!

Dr Gemma Newman has been a family doctor for 16 years. We developed the Happy Skin course with her.

Instagram: @plantpowerdoctor
https://gemmanewman.com/

Food

Your skin is often a reflection of the health of your internal organs – in particular, your liver and digestive system. Your liver is your body's 'sewage treatment plant'; one of its jobs is to deal with all the toxins and pollutants, so when your liver is not working optimally toxins can begin to filter through your other organs of elimination, such as your skin, which serves as 'back-up' for your liver. When toxins are eliminated through the skin, they may cause irritations such as rashes, pimples, blackheads and other skin conditions.

1. Antioxidants

A good analogy for oxidation is – imagine leaving your bike outside for months on end exposed to the elements. It starts to rust or 'oxidize', so a good way to think of antioxidants is that they stop you rusting! The main lifestyle factors that determine skin oxidation are smoking, drinking alcohol, not sleeping well, sun exposure, poor diet, pollutants and stress.

Along with a whole host of health benefits, antioxidants stop the premature ageing of our skin – they are wrinkle-fighters, pigmentation-tacklers and something that we need daily in our diets! The good news is that eating a wholefood plant-based diet is a great way of ensuring that you are getting plenty of antioxidants into your body, because they are most abundant in fruit and veg.

2. Essential fatty acids

Omega-3 essential fatty acids (EFAs) are vitally important for your skin and your body cannot make them itself. As you get older, your body struggles to retain moisture in its cells, so upping your EFA intake can help to counteract this. You won't see the benefits of drinking water in your skin unless you are getting your intake of EFAs, as without adequate omega-3s your skin can look dry and taut.

3. Fibre

There is no doubt that our gut health and our skin health are intrinsically linked – therefore, making sure we get enough fibre in our diet is key for skin health (see page 27 for more detail on fibre and gut health).

TIP

DAVE AND STEVE'S TOP TIPS FOR BOOSTING YOUR ANTIOXIDANT INTAKE:

- **Eat the rainbow.** The more brightly coloured a fruit or vegetable is, the more skin-loving antioxidants it contains. Aim to eat as many different coloured fruits and veggies as you can; this will also ensure that you get a wide variety of vitamins and minerals. It can be as easy as adding some red and yellow peppers to your stir-fry or adding beetroot to your hummus.

- **Bump up your berry intake.** Berries are super-high in antioxidants, particularly blueberries. Add some to your brekkie or have a few of them as a snack. They are super-low in calories too and can be fresh or frozen, depending on what is in season. Other beautiful berries include raspberries, strawberries and blackberries.

- **All hail kale.** Kale is one of the most nutritious green veggies on the planet. It's also packed with antioxidants – a perfect excuse to tuck into our kale crisps recipe in the snacks section (see page 254).

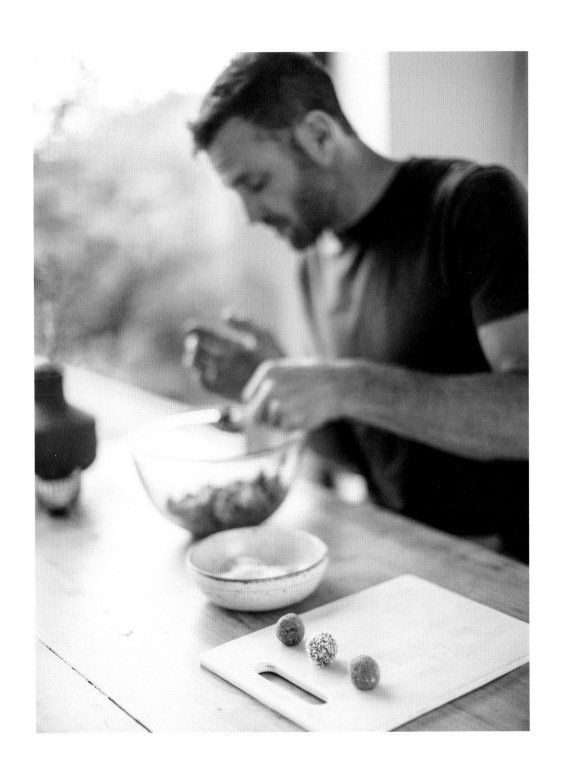

TIP

OUR TOP TIPS FOR GETTING MORE HEALTHY FATS INTO YOUR DIET:

- **Choose wholefood sources of fat**: (i.e. nuts, seeds, olives and avocados) over refined sources of fat such as oils (olive oil, coconut oil, sunflower oil, etc.). Our body needs a balance of omega-3 to omega-6. Refined oils are predominantly omega-6 EFA, and too much of these can inhibit our bodies' absorption of omega-3s, neutralizing skin-benefiting properties. These refined oils are found in most processed foods, including mayonnaise, pesto, baked goods and snack foods.

- **Eat some flax seeds and chia seeds.** These are both fantastic sources of essential fatty acids. Make some chia seed pudding (see page 130), or add milled flax seeds or whole chia seeds to porridge or dairy-free yoghurt for an extra boost of healthy fat. Ground flax seed stores for up to a month at room temperature and even longer in the fridge. (Flax seeds must be milled in order for them to be properly digested – you can mill flax seeds in a high-speed blender or coffee grinder, or just buy them in a supermarket pre-milled.)

- **Eat the healthiest nut of all.** Walnuts are one of the best sources of omega-3 EFA, so eat about 10–14 walnut halves for your daily omega-3s.

- **Make some of our tahini-rich hummus.** Tahini (blended sesame seed paste) is packed with goodness and healthy fats. It is a wholefood source of fat that unlike refined oils contains macronutrients other than simply fat. It is high in fat, so eat it in moderation. Enjoy it in our hummus (page 256), as a spread, or drizzle tahini with a small dash of maple syrup on antioxidant-rich fresh fruit for a tasty skin-loving snack!

TIP

OUR TOP TIPS FOR GETTING MORE FIBRE INTO YOUR DIET:

- **Eat your lentils and beans!** They are among the best sources of fibre in our diet. Fibre can only be found in plant-based foods – fruit, veg, beans, legumes and wholegrains. To instantly boost your fibre intake, add a tin of chickpeas or tinned lentils to your curry.

- **Eat green and yellow foods to reduce crow's feet.** In a study in Japan of 716 women to see the effects of diet on skin elasticity and the 'crow's feet' effect, researchers used the Daniell scale to determine the level of 'crow's feet' of each of the women – it's a scale of 1 to 6; 6 being the worst. The findings from the study were that a higher intake of green and yellow veg was associated with decreased facial wrinkling. Intake of saturated fat was found to be associated with more wrinkling.

- **Eat 'brown carbs'.** Replace all white carbohydrates, such as white pasta, white rice and white bread, with the wholegrain varieties. Wholegrain carbohydrates (i.e. brown rice, wholegrain pasta and wholemeal couscous) are great sources of fibre, and will help to keep you fuller for longer and keep your blood sugar levels more stable than white carbohydrates.

4. **Avoid processed foods**

If your skin had a number-one nemesis it would be refined and processed foods that are high in sugar.

They can deplete your good bacteria: These refined foods are high in sugar, and this sugar feeds the 'bad' bacteria in your gut. If you have an unhealthy gut it can have a big impact on your overall health and especially on the appearance of your skin, including spots, inflammation, eczema and rosacea. This is why many skin-supportive regimes start with eating fibre-rich foods that feed your healthy bacteria. If you want to learn more about gut health, check out our Happy Gut section (see page 80). It's all about building up your gut health, which of course is linked to skin health.

They can cause excess oil production, leading to oilier skin: When you eat processed foods, your body releases large amounts of insulin into your bloodstream to absorb the excess sugar into your cells. When lots of insulin is dumped into your blood, research shows that sebum (oil) is also produced and can lead to clogged pores, which may lead to pimples, whiteheads and blackheads.

Processed foods AGE your skin: They literally age your skin by producing AGEs (advanced glycation end products). When you eat refined carbs and processed foods such as white bread, the refined sugars attach themselves to proteins in your body such as collagen (which is linked to healthy, plump robust skin), forming new molecules which are called AGEs – these are non-reversible, meaning that some of your skin-smoothing collagen is lost for ever.

Fast food, meats and processed meats: Fast food and processed meats are high in omega-6s and saturated fat, both of which cause inflammation in the body. Inflammation is at the root of many skin conditions, so cutting out or dramatically reducing pro-inflammatory foods such as fast foods and processed meats makes loads of sense in terms of happy skin. Red meat in particular is linked to inflammation. Also consumption of all types of meat has been shown to increase C-reactive protein, which is a marker used to measure the level of inflammation in our bodies.

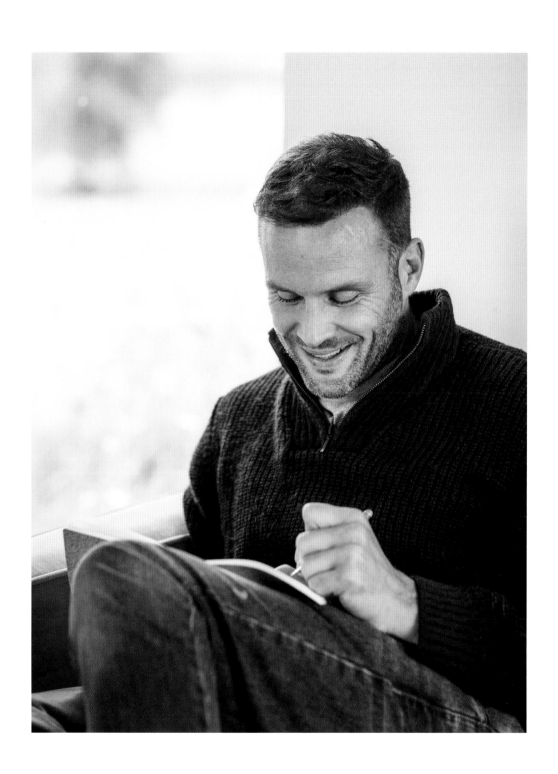

Happy Skin diary

The Happy Skin course is a way to improve the foundational aspects of your health, which are reflected through your skin. Healthy skin starts from within. As well as our recipes and meal plans, we have a diary template for you (see opposite) – it's a great way to track your sleep, your exercise levels, your water intake, your stress levels, as well as the foods you eat. This serves as a great tool to keep track of the essential elements that will result in your Happy Skin: recording all your good work will help keep you on track and over time will show you how consistent you have been. Insights will start to emerge and it will help show you just how powerful lifestyle changes can be on your skin.

"

Skin has always been problematic for me. Since turning 30 I've decided to invest in my skin and learn how to better protect and look after it going forward.

The Happy Skin course is just brilliant! From an abundance of interesting and easy-to-follow recipes, to expert advice from leading professionals, and online support and accountability that spurs you on, it does cover all of the bases on good skin health.

For me, one of the biggest lessons I learnt is that I have been treating my skin incorrectly. Who knew I have oily, dehydrated skin? The skin diary, 'skin saver' homework, weekly quizzes and live Q&As were all great tools in helping me discover this.

I'm drinking more water, prioritizing my sleep, and I'm mindful of what I am putting into my body as well as what I am putting on to my skin. SPF and double cleansing are my new best friends, and sea swims are a weekly occurrence. Two months on and I'm still reaping the benefits thanks to Dave and Steve!

Cooking is no longer a chore, and looking after my skin is now a habit. I am not only more confident in the kitchen, but more confident in myself.

"

– *Lynsey*

HAPPY SKIN DIARY TEMPLATE

Please tick the box if:

- You have eaten your Happy Skin meals INSIDE
- You applied your skincare regime OUTSIDE
- If applicable, you applied minimal makeup ON TOP
- Number of litres of WATER consumed
- Give yourself a number between 1 and 10 to reflect STRESS levels
- Did you eat refined SUGAR?
- Please list how many hours of SLEEP you had
- Have you included ME TIME in your day?
- Please list how many hours of DAYLIGHT you had

	Monday	Tuesday	Wednesday	Thursday	Friday	Saturday	Sunday
Inside							
Outside							
On Top							
Water							
Stress							
Sugar/Diet							
Sleep							
Me Time							
Daylight							
Additional Comments							

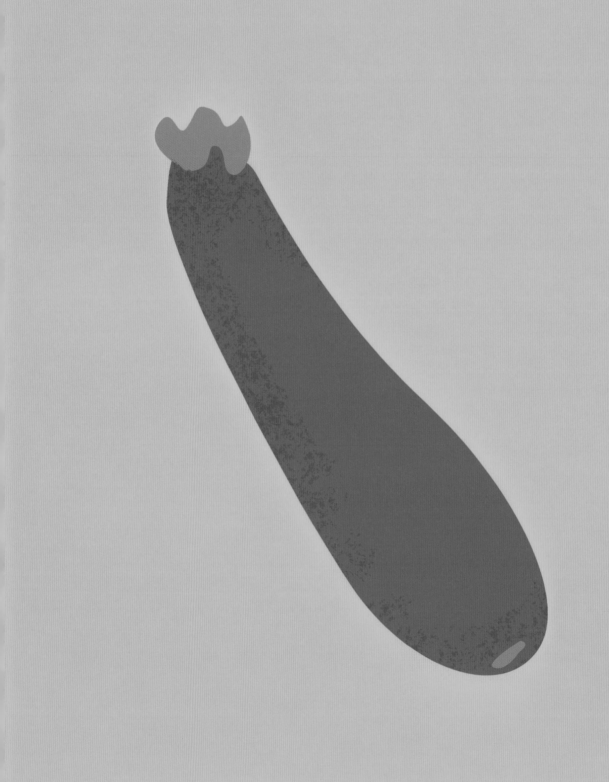

Chapter 5

Happy Shape

Want to reach your Happy Shape with no portion control, no calorie-counting and all-you-can-eat delicious tasty food? Sounds like a dream come true, right? Welcome to Happy Shape, a plan that has helped thousands of people become more confident and happy with their body.

We all want to feel confident and comfortable in our bodies, to fit into those jeans that represent our Happy Shape and not have to wrestle them on, to hold our head high and feel confident in our body as we walk down the street knowing that we look and feel great. Happy Shape is about making this feeling a reality. It's not a diet or a quick fix; it's about forming the simple habits that will have a positive effect on your life as well as on your waistline. Being overweight in the vast majority of cases is more than simply excess body fat. It is very often a representation of poor lifestyle habits. Happy Shape is about getting to the root of why you might be carrying excess weight and building a foundation for you to recalibrate your health and relationship to your body so that you gain more energy, sleep better, have better moods, become more confident and are happy with your shape. This may sound like a big promise, but bear with us – let's go one step at a time.

"

Over 8 weeks I lost 24lb and have never felt better. Two days into the new lifestyle I had major withdrawals from all of the junk and sugar I had been eating, on the third day it was like a switch! I felt so happy and positive, my skin improved, my metabolic age and my visceral fat reading all decreased and I had so much more energy.

It is an easy plan to follow and the recipes are absolutely delicious. Each meal is so well planned and some of them transported me back to my childhood. The Happy Pear know their flavours and so many of their meals do feel like a belly hug!

Making a move to a plant-based lifestyle has had such a positive impact on my life and I was also amazed at the savings I made on my shopping trips from changing to a plant-based diet.

"

– Cliodhna

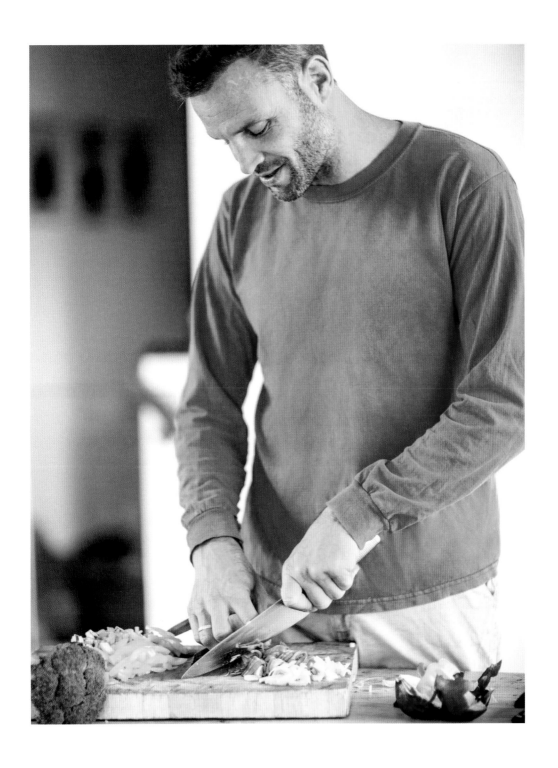

Benefits of the Happy Shape plan

- **More energy:** Plant-based foods are oxygen-rich, high in water and low in saturated fat, so will help optimize your blood flow and pump all the nutrients around your body – along with getting your steps in and doing our workouts, your mitochondria (the energy powerhouses of your cells) will be bouncing with energy!

- **Better moods:** Wholefoods are high in complex carbohydrates, and also avoiding refined and processed foods will mean you have a more steady, even release of energy throughout the day.

- **Feeling lighter:** Happy Shape is built on high-fibre wholefoods that are naturally low in calories – you will be feeling fuller, eating more, yet losing weight!

- **Better sleep:** More movement, better food, more self-care and a focus on forming decent sleep habits will lead to much more consistent restful sleep (see page 38 for more on sleep).

- **Better digestion:** Whole plant-based foods are prebiotics and feed the healthy bacteria in your gut, aiding your digestion. Cutting out refined foods will help colonize the healthy strains of microorganisms in your gut, leading to better digestion, among many other benefits.

- **More confidence in your body:** It's a self-fulfilling virtuous cycle, when you are making better food choices, making time for getting your steps in, giving yourself some 'me time' – your confidence levels will start to soar, your self-love will grow, you will feel more proud and happy in your own skin and all this will further spur you on!

- **Sustained healthy weight loss or maintenance:** Happy Shape will help you to lose weight, and the massive positive side-effects will encourage and inspire you to keep it up so that it becomes your new norm.

Since entering my fifties I have found that not only has my shape changed, but it seems much harder to shift the pounds, so I was looking for something different but sustainable. I am home a lot, as I work freelance, so I enjoyed trying out the new recipes every day.

The recipes are very straightforward, and many can be made using storecupboard ingredients and fresh vegetables. Within a few days of starting the plan I felt lighter, less bloated, and I was delighted that everyone in the house was enjoying the food. Before the programme, I would regularly feel tired around 2 or 3 o'clock and reach for the tea and biscuits to give me a boost. However, by day 4 of the plan I noticed that the afternoon slump was gone.

The plan encourages you to track your steps. I usually take our dog, Rusky, for a walk every day but I was shocked when I started to track my steps, to see that I was getting way less than the recommended 10,000 steps a day. So I started adding another walk to my day without the dog and gradually built up to 10,000 steps most days. This has stuck with me and it now feels odd if I don't get up and out for my steps.

I did lose weight and still have more to go, but I have more energy and feel much more positive about achieving my goal!

– *Ruth*

Energy density

The Happy Shape plan is built on low energy density foods. Energy density is the amount of calories per weight of food. Lower energy density foods provide fewer calories per gram of food – this means that you can have satisfying portions of these foods with a relatively low calorie content. They are high in water and fibre, neither of which have calories and both of which bulk up foods, adding volume and mass to them without calories.

We all tend to eat the same amount of food each day – approximately 2kg. By choosing low energy dense foods it makes it a lot easier to lose weight or maintain a healthy weight.

- **Low energy density foods = less than 1.5 kcal/g**
  This includes most fruit and veg, particularly the highest in water such as undressed salad leaves, asparagus, broccoli, berries, cauliflower, peppers, mushrooms and onions, to name a few.

- **Medium energy density foods = 1.5 to 4 kcal/g**
  Beans and legumes, cooked starchy veg and wholegrains all fall into this category, as do plant milks, tofu and tempeh.

- **High energy density foods = more than 4 kcal/g**
  These tend to have a low water content and as a result tend to be higher in fat and calories – most refined and processed foods fit in this category, as they are high in refined oils. The only whole plant-based foods that are high energy density are nuts, seeds, olives, avocados, nut butters and tahini. If weight loss is your goal, we recommend you try to minimize these and limit your intake to a small handful of nuts (see page 98 for details) and to avoid nut butter or seed butters, as they are too difficult to eat only a teaspoon at a time!

All the Happy Shape recipes (marked with ◯) and the meal plan on page 114 are low in energy density, so when we mean eat as much as you want, we genuinely mean it. All the food will fill you up and sustain you while also being low in calories.

I have been vegan for 11 years, but over the years the weight has piled on. When I started out, most of my meals were cooked from scratch using good ingredients, but as more and more processed vegan foods came on the market my weight and health began to suffer. Although I stopped smoking at the same time I went vegan, recently I was diagnosed with mild chronic obstructive pulmonary disease (COPD) and raised cholesterol levels (my family have a history of heart problems), and to keep myself well for the future, I decided it was time for a change. It is very scary being diagnosed with what could be a life-limiting disease, but my research showed how weight, diet and exercise are very important.

I started following the Happy Pear on YouTube and I loved that their recipes were quick, easy to follow and made with readily recognizable ingredients. Every recipe I tried was delicious. I started the Happy Shape Club and was delighted to lose 12lb in the first 3 weeks. I feel so much better in myself, I have no more bloating, my skin has improved and, best of all, I have tons of new-found energy!

The plan is very easy to follow and all mapped out for you. I was the original couch potato but now I am brisk walking for 30 minutes a day on top of a daily workout.

My breathing has improved so much that my doctor halved my inhaled steroid medication and I fully expect my cholesterol count to go down at my next blood test. I certainly feel a lot more confident about my future prospects with COPD and being able to live life to the full and enjoy my grandchildren for many years to come.

99

– *Frances*

The science

The perfect diet for a lifetime of sustained healthy weight is one that:

- **Fills you up** and doesn't leave you feeling hungry or deprived.
- **Leaves you feeling full** for longer.
- **Tastes delicious** and has lots of variety.
- **Nourishes you** with vitamins and minerals.
- **Is high in fibre.**
- **Is low in calories.**
- **Has the side-effects of improved energy,** better digestion, better moods and more focus, to name a few!

The wholefood plant-based diet in our Happy Shape meal plan ticks every one of these boxes.

FIBRE

Increasing the amount of fibre-rich foods you eat could be the best piece of advice for weight loss. Studies have shown that if the average person in the UK increased their fibre intake by 14g to reach the RDA (recommended daily allowance) they would consume 10% fewer calories every day. There are many reasons that eating more fibre reduces overall calorie intake:

- **Fibre bulks up your food** while not adding calories.
- **It has no calories**, it's an indigestible bulking agent made of plant cellulose that passes right through you.
- **Foods that are high in fibre typically take longer to chew**, meaning more hormones are released to signal satiation.
- **It fills up your stomach**, signalling satiation.
- **Due to fibre's indigestible nature** we can rarely absorb all the nutrition from high-fibre foods, meaning some of the calories are out of the equation as they end up being flushed down the toilet!

(See page 27 for more on fibre and its benefits.)

PLANT-BASED FOODS ARE HIGH IN WATER

Like fibre, water adds volume and mass to foods without adding calories. You could eat a handful of raisins or you could eat a handful of grapes – same food, but which has more calories? The raisins do: the grapes per weight are about 80% water, so 80% of their weight has no calories! In a famous experiment published in the *European Journal of Nutrition*,* dozens of foods were tested for their ability to satiate appetite, and the high water content in the food was the number-one factor that filled you up.

Water alongside a meal is not the same as water inside a food, because of a concept known as 'sieving'. When water is consumed alongside a meal your stomach just siphons off the water and 'sieves' it off the solid food. Whereas water that is part of a food empties more slowly from your stomach over time – that's why blended soup is in fact more filling than chunky soup. Interesting, eh!

* https://pubmed.ncbi.nlm.nih.gov/7498104/

NOT ALL CALORIES ARE CREATED EQUAL

The food industry wants you to believe that the source of our calories doesn't matter, that in fact a calorie of chocolate is the same as a calorie of apple, but this is definitely not the case. In his book *How Not to Diet*, Dr Michael Greger gives a brilliant example: 240 calories of coke versus 240 calories of carrots (10 carrots).

In a tightly controlled laboratory setting these two foods would be equal in terms of calories, but in the real world this is definitely not the case. You can chug a bottle of coke in 1 minute, but to eat 240 calories of carrots would take more than 2½ hours of sustained constant chewing. Not only would your jaw get sore, you might not even be able to fit them in – 240 calories of carrots is about 10 average carrots, weighing about 610g. Carrots, like all whole plant foods, are high in fibre, which bulks up your food but has no calories. What is more, you wouldn't even be able to eat all the calories, as some bits of vegetable matter will pass right through you straight into the toilet bowl without being absorbed; a calorie may be a calorie but not if it ends up in the toilet bowl!

All calories are not created equal. Try to get your calories from whole plant foods, as these will fill you up and nourish your body in a way that refined and processed foods never will.

66

I started my Happy Pear journey after having my second child. I had a rough pregnancy and still managed to gain a significant amount of weight! I had suffered with hyperemesis and because of this couldn't cook because of the smell of food and so had gotten into very bad habits with eating just to survive. I first did the Happy Heart course and was shocked at how much weight I lost but also how much healthier I became!

The Happy Shape Club has totally turned my life around. I have struggled with postnatal depression and have found it difficult to motivate myself to do anything. Now, I am a happier, healthier, more positive version of myself!

I love exercise, which is something I hadn't done in a long while. I am more attuned to my body's needs; I make all my meals myself. I have also learnt to slow down and to relax and take a breath, so I can watch what is going on around me instead of being dragged along by life.

99

– Louise

EXERCISE VS DIET?

As a general rule your weight is 80% down to what you eat and only 20% down to your level of exercise, assuming you are not an elite athlete! It is far easier to consume fewer calories than it is to burn them off, but there is more to it, which we will explain.

Eating fewer calories is definitely the quickest and easiest way to start shedding the pounds, because with the right food it's relatively easy to cut the calories without feeling deprived. Once you have learnt how to prepare delicious, healthy meals from this book which are low in calories, you will start to lose weight without feeling constantly hungry.

Exercise does have a part to play – when we increase the amount of physical activity we do, this of course burns more calories, but it also increases our resting metabolic rate, which means we burn more calories even when we are not exercising.

Just to give a bit of context, if you exercise for 30 minutes the average calories you will burn are:

	Woman (70kg)	Man (80kg)
Light jogging	205 cals	244 cals
Weightlifting	112 cals	133 cals
Yoga	120 cals	178 cals
Cycling (moderately)	260 cals	311 cals
HIIT session (high intensity interval training)	372 cals	444 cals

An average banana is about 100 calories, so for 30 minutes of jogging you will burn nearly 2 bananas or 1 Mars bar (230 calories), and for 30 minutes of yoga you will burn approximately 1 can of coke (140 calories).

I have had such a great time learning to follow a true vegan, unprocessed diet. I loved how the lads called it a culinary adventure, as that is what it was. The course had easy-to-follow recipes, using vegetables that I had honestly never used before and which made the most amazing and delicious meals. The biggest change was the goal of 10,000 steps a day, but I did it and enjoyed myself. I finished the 12-week journey and have lost 20lb. I enjoy who I have become: healthy, motivated and moving!

– Jennifer

SMART GOALS, BY DR SUE KENNEALLY

You are more likely to succeed with your weight-loss efforts if you have a clear plan of not just where you want to get to, but how and why. The most important of these is why.

Having a clear reason why you want to lose weight is key to your endeavours, so whether it's to get rid of your aches and pains, or your doctor has advised you that it's necessary, or if you just want to look hot, or whatever, get that firmly in your mind to get you through the times when you face temptation to give up.

When it comes to setting goals, we often talk about SMART goals, which means Specific, Measurable, Achievable, Relevant and Time-specific.

- Specific – instead of saying 'I'm going to get more active', you specify that this means: 'I'm going to start walking for 30 minutes every day at lunchtime.'
- Measurable – you can only change what you can measure, so make it about a number of servings of fruits and veggies, or minutes of physical activity.
- Achievable – make it something that stretches you, but if it's completely out of reach this could actually make things worse, because you will have to deal with the negativity of failure.
- Relevant – it does have to be something that should actually result in weight loss!
- Time-specific – give yourself a date to achieve it by, but don't beat yourself up if you don't quite make it.

You are likely to get better results if you don't make your goals about the number on the scales, but instead give yourself challenges that are likely to result in weight loss. So instead of 'I'm going to lose some weight', make your goal 'I'm going to eat more fruits and vegetables', or 'I'm going to get more active.'

An example of a SMART goal would be: 'I'm going to increase my fruit and vegetable intake by eating a banana with my breakfast and eating carrot sticks and hummus for my mid-morning snack instead of crisps, starting on Monday.'

Lastly, write your goal down and put it somewhere where you will see it regularly. People who write their goals down are far more likely to achieve them than those who don't. It may also help to write it down in the present tense, so instead of 'I am going to go to my favourite gym class every Tuesday', write it as 'I go to my favourite gym class every Tuesday.'

Check out our SMART pull-out goal sheet on our website. We recommend you fill this in and put it somewhere where you see it daily as a great source of motivation and inspiration.

Dr Sue Kenneally, MBBS, MRCGP, MSc (NutMed), ANutr, is co-founder of the British Society of Lifestyle Medicine. She sits on the board of Plant-Based Health Professionals UK and is SCOPE certified in obesity management, working with the University of South Wales in the study of weight management. We developed the Happy Shape course with Dr Sue.
Instagram: @plantbasedlifestylemedic
http://drsuekenneally.com/

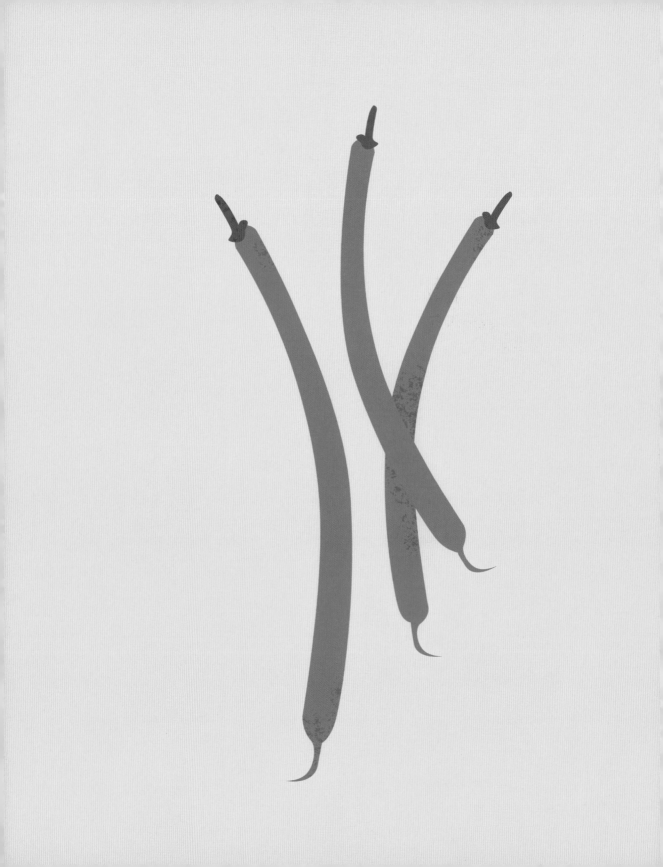

Chapter 6

Happy Gut

The Happy Gut plan will help you dramatically improve your digestive health and microbiome as well as so many other positive side-effects – like better mood, glowing skin and more energy. It is rooted in science and has helped tens of thousands of people improve their health.

Thousands of years ago, Hippocrates, the father of medicine, said, 'All disease begins in the gut.' Our experience with thousands of people on our online Happy Gut course makes us agree. From a recent survey of the participants:

- **98%** would recommend to a friend.
- **84%** with bloating improved their health.
- **89%** with IBS reported improved gut health.
- **75%** improved their gut health.
- **44%** improved their mood.
- **43%** improved their energy.

Here are some fascinating facts about the gut which show how important gut health is to your health and wellbeing:

- **Tens of trillions of bacteria and microorganisms** (that is 10 with 14 zeros after it!), existing mostly in our small intestine, make up our 'microbiome'.
- **70% of our immune system cells** are based in our gut.
- **There is a very important nerve**, called the vagus nerve, that transfers information directly from our gut to our brain, meaning that the health of our gut is very likely to impact our moods, the foods we crave, our concentration and our mental health.
- **The richest microbiomes ever recorded** were those of the Yanomami tribe in the Amazon jungle, who had had no previous contact with the modern world. Traditional societies tend to have more diverse microbiomes in general, and the key is thought to be their extraordinary fibre intake, which can reach 120g a day, nearly eight times the UK and Irish average.

Being a working mother of two little ones under the age of 3, I have to be very organized for my work week and LOVE the meal plans, shopping lists and recipes!

– Danielle

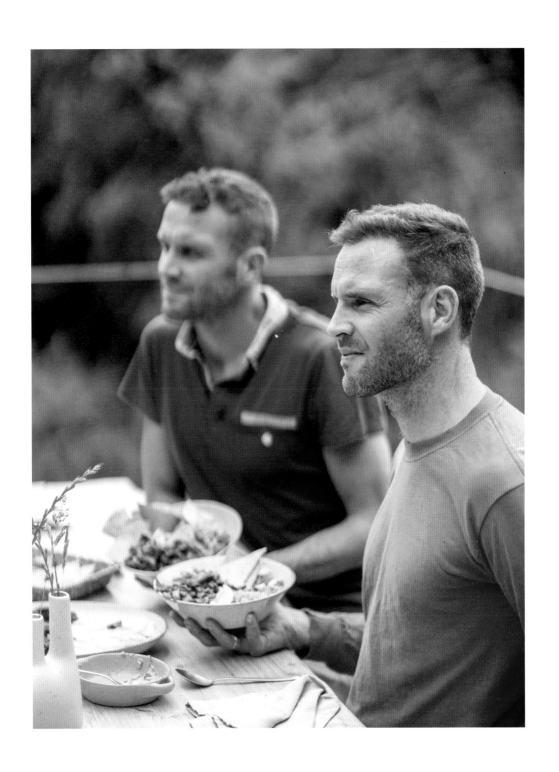

Through our online Happy Gut course we have learnt that the single most important factor for influencing the health of your gut is what you eat. And which foods do you think make the healthy bacteria strains thrive and grow in numbers? You guessed it, it's fibre-rich plant foods! Fibre is only found in fruit, veg, beans, legumes, wholegrains, and nuts and seeds. Animal foods and refined foods do not contain any fibre. In fact, fibre is a prebiotic to our microbiome, it is the food that our bacteria and microorganisms feed on and it helps to encourage them to be healthy and flourish, which in turn improves our physical and mental health.

In the UK and Ireland, 9 out of 10 people get only about half their recommended daily allowance (RDA) of fibre, meaning they are not eating enough fruit, veg, beans, lentils and wholegrains. The minimum RDA of fibre is about 30g. If you follow our Happy Gut meal plan on page 118 you'll be getting at least 45g of fibre a day, while also following a low-FODMAP diet (see page 90 for more on FODMAPs).

About 2 years ago my entire immune system seemed to collapse and I developed around 6 autoimmune conditions overnight. I had severe difficulty in breathing, even standing up was enough to put me out of breath. I developed numerous skin conditions, one being extreme pain and sensitivity to anything touching my skin, even the feel of clothing on my skin was painful. I had zero energy, constantly felt as if I was in a permanent state of exhaustion and suffered with pounding headaches and nausea. As if all of this wasn't enough, I also developed rheumatoid arthritis in my right hand.

In the search for answers, I went to countless doctors both in Ireland and the UK who, frustratingly, had no answers whatsoever for me. I struggled to find a doctor who would look at where these conditions were coming from as opposed to simply treating the symptoms. I eventually found a functional doctor who diagnosed me with dysbiosis, which is a microbial imbalance in the gut. This apparently caused my immune system to collapse and my body to start attacking itself.

I then came across the Happy Gut course and I knew it was just the answer I was looking for to rebuild my gut and start getting my health back. The thought of going vegan petrified me, as I didn't even know how to make toast, let alone cook a meal from scratch! I knew that giving up milk, chocolate and cheese was going to be incredibly tough; however, I was willing to go 'cold-tofu', as my health was more important than anything else.

After I followed the first few recipes and produced food that blew my socks off with taste, I began to get excited about food for the first time in my life! My diet used to be very processed and bland, and everything I ate came from a packet, with the same food being eaten all the time. Now, I eat a huge variety of fruits and vegetables in the most amazing dishes every single day and I can't wait for my next meal.

A year later, I have made a full recovery from every symptom with the exception of arthritis, which I am still working on. I couldn't be happier with the new direction my life has taken and this love for fresh wholefood is something I will never change.

– Peter

THE HAPPY GUT COURSE, BY DR ALAN DESMOND

Working on the Happy Gut course with Steve, Dave and Rosie was an absolute pleasure. At times it seemed like every planning meeting started with fresh coffee, breakfast, a swim in the sea, second breakfast and a yoga session followed by great conversation. But there was some serious work to do too. The 'FODMAP process' has been shown to be very effective in clinical trials, with a 70–80% success rate in treating people with IBS-type symptoms. One of our main obstacles was that FODMAPs are inherently healthy substances that help your gut microbiome to thrive and produce beneficial compounds including short-chain fatty acids. Wholegrains, garlic, onions, avocados, apples and mangoes are some of my favourite foods and they are all high in FODMAPs. Unhealthy foods like steak, eggs and bacon are naturally free of FODMAPs and often feature in traditional low-FODMAP recipes.

We set ourselves a challenge: to build an online course that was as effective as the existing FODMAP process but used healthy ingredients from the start. We wanted the Happy Gut course to be available to people with coeliac disease. The task was to design an eating plan built on recipes that were healthy, wholefood, plant-based, low in fermentable ingredients and gluten-free. We also needed to design a system to reintroduce all those healthy foods and wholegrains in the space of 6 weeks. And the recipes had to be tasty and easy to prepare!

Steve, Dave, Rosie and I were in Pearville to launch the course. It was all very exciting! Our first Happy Gut Heroes started in early January 2019. Within weeks, hundreds of individuals around the world were trying out the plan. It became apparent that the Happy Gut community was a mix of people with known IBS or IBS-type symptoms, people with other gut health issues and people who just wanted to learn more about the gut microbiome while enjoying new plant-based recipes. After a few months we paused to evaluate the outcomes. We had certainly disproved the theory that the FODMAP process had to be unhealthy. Using our high-fibre meal plans, packed with a variety of plants, we had achieved success rates to equal those seen in the traditional clinical setting: 89% of Happy Gut Heroes who signed up to improve IBS-type symptoms reported success, and 98% said that they would recommend the course to a friend.

As a consultant gastroenterologist, I know that a wholefood plant-based diet ticks all the right boxes for optimal gut health and overall health. Continuing to support our Happy Gut community while knowing that we have already helped thousands of people to make the switch to a plant-based diet while improving their digestive health has become one of the highlights of my working week!

Dr Alan Desmond's 5 keys to improving your gut health

1. **Adopt a wholefood plant-based diet:** Try to base your diet around fruits, veg, beans, legumes and wholegrains and cut out or dramatically minimize refined and animal foods. (See Chapter 1 for more on this.)

2. **Exercise and move more:** Research shows that those who exercise and move more have healthier microbiomes than those who do not. (See page 34 for more on this.)

3. **Get your sleep:** Sleep greatly affects our microbiome: it turns out that our microorganisms, like us, thrive with a good sleep routine. (See page 38 for more on this.)

4. **Spend time outdoors:** Research suggests that spending time in nature exposes us to different microorganisms that further strengthen the diversity and health of our microbiome. If you can spend time in different

ecosystems, even better – forests, parks, seaside, mountains, etc.

5. **Avoid antibiotics, if you can:** Antibiotics save so many lives every day in cases where they are needed, but when not necessary try to avoid them, as they will have a significant negative effect on your gut health.

Dr Alan Desmond, MB BCh, BMedSc, MRCPI, FRCP, is a consultant gastroenterologist and author of The Plant-Based Diet Revolution. Dr Desmond was central to developing the Happy Gut course and has also been involved in the Happy Heart course. He actively promotes a wholefood plant-based diet, particularly for patients with chronic digestive disorders.
Instagram: @dr.alandesmond

The reason behind why I chose this course initially was to help my symptoms of IBS and stomach discomfort. The course has dramatically changed my relationship with food and my outlook on health. Within the first week my symptoms have dramatically decreased. The Happy Gut course has enabled me to eat a wide variety of healthy plant-based food that I would have never tried previously. The course has changed the way I look at food – I no longer get anxious around mealtimes about how my body will react to foods, the step-by-step low-FODMAP meal plan makes cooking exciting again and I now look forward to trying new foods. My sole benefit of doing the course was to improve my digestive health, but I have gained so much more, I have built up a knowledge of how the microbiome works, I feel I can cook tasty plant-based foods and I have connected with a wide community of like-minded people. So far my experience with the Happy Gut course has exceeded all my expectations and been the best investment for my health and wellbeing.

– Orla

I feel mentally and physically lighter and stronger after the Happy Gut course. From the gut reset all the way through the reintroductions, I felt my digestion went from strength to strength. I have more energy, and the recovery time from jet lag has diminished by many factors. On the course I found the knowledge, tools, community and motivation to plan, source and prepare the best possible food. I'm absolutely delighted I joined. I know I will be reaping the benefits for the rest of my life.

– George

FODMAPS, BY DIETITIAN ROSIE MARTIN

Supporting people with an unhappy gut makes up a substantial part of my day-to-day work as a dietitian. Through supporting people with digestive issues, I have witnessed the dramatic impact diet and lifestyle can have, not just on someone's gut health and symptoms, but on their ability to carry out everyday activities and enjoy their life. Through my dietetic clinics, I also see the dramatic effect that a low-FODMAP diet plan can have when nothing else seems to help. The low-FODMAP diet is a short-term plan allowing individuals to identify which specific fermentable carbohydrates (FODMAP) impact their symptoms, and enable them to take back control of their gut health long-term using the valuable information they have gained. FODMAP is an acronym which stands for 'Fermentable Oligo-saccharides, Di-saccharides, Mono-saccharides and Polyols'.

Within healthcare, dietitians only use a strict low-FODMAP diet when other potential causes of symptoms have been ruled out, e.g. coeliac disease or IBD (inflammatory bowel disease). This is important so that nothing more serious is missed. Through working in plant-based food and nutrition, however, Steve, Dave, Dr Alan and myself have all been amazed at the vast number of stories we have heard from people struggling with gut issues when moving to predominantly, or exclusively, plant-based foods. Switching to a wholefood plant-based diet can dramatically increase the levels of both fibre and FODMAPs in the diet; this is very healthy for our friendly gut microbiota, which thrive on these foods, but can lead to an array of short-term symptoms including bloating, flatulence, abdominal pain, and loose stools or constipation (or both!).

In the Happy Gut meal plan (see page 118) all the recipes are low-FODMAP, and the 6-week programme will help guide you through the diet (see page 93). Week 1 is a gut reset week, and then through each of the following 5 weeks we slowly reintroduce FODMAPs one at a time so that it is easy for you to gauge your sensitivities to each one.

If you are struggling to beat the bloat and don't want to follow our 6-week approach, it's a good idea to build at least some of your meals in a FODMAP-controlled manner. Most cookbooks do not take this important issue into account. Garlic, onions, cashew nuts, chickpeas and lentils are all healthy choices, but are also all high in FODMAPs. Many plant-based recipes use these foods in significant quantities, often in combination! All the Happy Gut recipes with the ⊜ icon are low-FODMAP, so will be easy on your digestion, while also being high in fibre.

Rosie Martin is a registered dietitian working within the NHS, with a special interest in disease prevention and plant-based nutrition. Rosie helped develop the Happy Gut and Happy Shape courses with us.
Instagram: @plantdietitianrosie

Our Happy Gut 6-week process

HOW TO REINTRODUCE FODMAPS

Reintroducing FODMAPs is a crucial part of the plan, and we don't recommend anyone stays on a low-FODMAP diet for a long period of time, even if you have seen a dramatic improvement in symptoms.

Each week you will be reintroducing one FODMAP back into your diet. To do this, add a portion of your chosen high-FODMAP food to your Happy Gut low-FODMAP meals. You will increase the number of portions you add over 4 days to identify your tolerance level.

Complete your reintroductions each week in the following way:

- **Monday** – 1 portion with lunch
- **Tuesday** – 1 portion with lunch + 1 portion with dinner
- **Wednesday** – 2 portions with lunch + 1 portion with dinner
- **Thursday** – 2 portions with lunch + 2 portions with dinner

For example, in week 2 you could add 4 tablespoons of Happy Gut hummus (see page 256) to your Happy Gut high protein quinoa salad (see page 185). In week 3 you could add half an avocado to the top of your Asian broccoli salad, and add sugar snap peas in week 4. In week 5 you might brighten up your high protein quinoa salad with pomegranate seeds, spring onions or crushed almonds. In week 6, why not add 2 slices of wholewheat toast to your lentil sambar soup!

If you experience excess bloating, gas or digestive discomfort, you have identified that your gut microbiome may be sensitive to the higher intake of the FODMAP you are testing. Make a note of the number of portions you managed symptom-free prior to this, and stop the reintroduction. At this point, wait until your symptoms have settled before commencing the next reintroduction week.

It is important to make sure after each reintroduction, even if you tolerated the food, to remove it from your diet before commencing the next reintroduction. FODMAPs have a cumulative effect, so you should keep your underlying diet low-FODMAP for each reintroduction week to work out your specific sensitivities.

At the end of the 6 weeks, you will have an awareness of any foods that you are more sensitive to.

Week 1: gut reset week (you can extend this for up to 4 weeks)

Choose from the Happy Gut recipes, which are all low-FODMAP and marked with ⊜ . Use the Happy Gut meal plan and shopping list (see pages 118–21) to make it easier.

Week 2: reintroducing galacto-oligosaccharides (carbohydrates found in beans and legumes)

A single portion of this FODMAP can be made up with any of the following:

- 105g black beans
- 75g peas
- 88g haricot beans
- 90g split peas (boiled)

Week 3: reintroducing polyols (naturally occurring sugars in certain veg – avocados, peaches, sweet potatoes, etc.)

A single portion of this FODMAP can be made up of any of the following:

- ½ an avocado (80g)
- 160g blackberries
- 96g coconut
- 1 medium peach (145g)
- 2 apricots (70g)
- 75g cauliflower
- 2 stalks of celery (75g)
- 100g sweet potato

Week 4: reintroducing fructose – a fruit sugar

A single portion of this FODMAP can be made up of any of the following:

- 1 medium fresh fig (50g)
- ½ a mango (140g)
- 25 sugar snap peas (75g)

Week 5: reintroducing non-grain fructans (alliums – onions and garlic)

A single portion of this FODMAP can be made up of any of the following:

- 1 clove of garlic (3g)
- 1 spring onion/scallion (32g)
- 1 shallot (6g)
- 1 grapefruit (207g)
- seeds from 1 small pomegranate (87g)
- 2 tablespoons dried cranberries (30g)
- 2 tablespoons raisins (26g)
- 20 cashew nuts (30g)
- 2 tablespoons tahini (40g)

Week 6: reintroducing wholegrain fructans/ gluten-free equivalents

A single portion of this FODMAP can be made up with any of the following:

- 2 slices of wholegrain wheat bread (52g)
- 148g wholewheat pasta (cooked)
- 154g wholemeal couscous (cooked)
- 225g pearl barley (cooked)

Week 6: Gluten-free option

- 2 slices of your favourite gluten-free bread
- 2 bonus slices of our gluten-free porridge bread (see page 134)
- An extra half portion of any of the meals you are enjoying in this week's meal plan

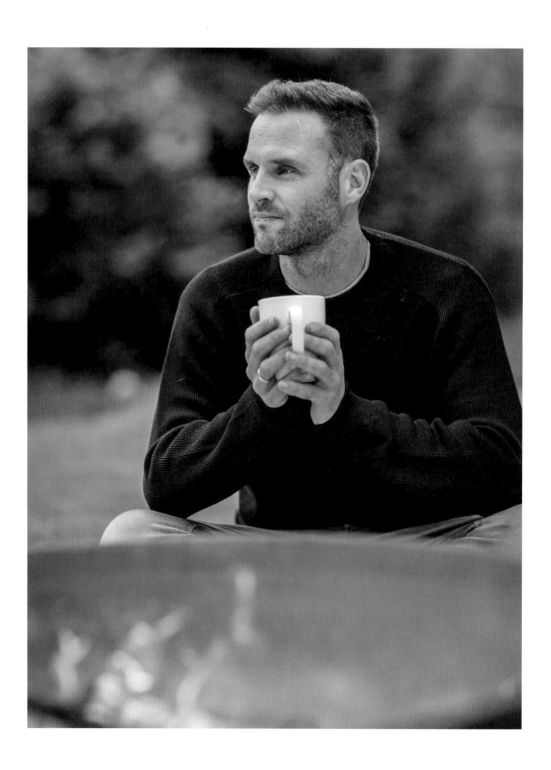

66

I was down a jean size after 8 days of the course and they're getting looser each week :). I've had bloating for 30 years. This is the first time I have had 90% reduction of symptoms while eating 3 meals a day. At other times I had no symptoms because I was eating next to nothing. I think the main point for me is the Happy Gut course gives me a way of life where I'm feeling healthy and therefore in balance with life. Head fog has gone, joint pain reduced, bloating 90% gone, mood stable, fluid retention hugely reduced. I was so unwell last winter there was a suggestion of fibromyalgia which led me here – with a 9-year-old I can't be sick! My almost-18-year-old has given up cows' milk and is eating more plant-based too.

99

– Janet

66

Last year, I was diagnosed with small intestinal bacterial overgrowth (SIBO) and advised to follow a low-FODMAP diet.

I struggled to follow the diet on my own, so I was thrilled to discover the Happy Gut course. I have learnt so much about nutrition and healthy eating from following the plan and my gut issues have greatly improved.

I would highly recommend the Happy Gut course to anyone who has an un-happy gut!

99

– Irene

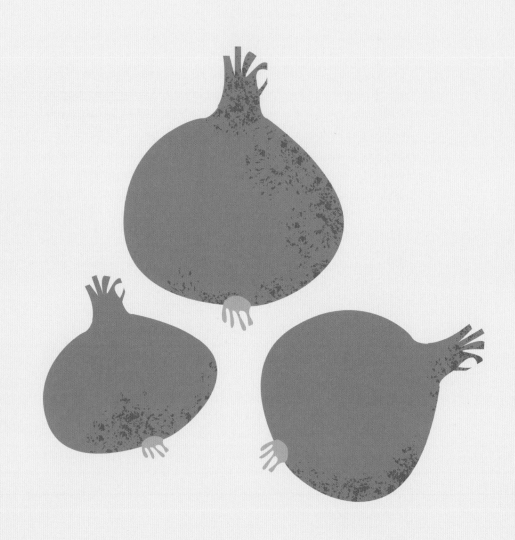

Chapter 7

Meal Plans

This is a really practical chapter with label reading (a skill we highly recommend you develop), what storecupboard staples we use as well as 4 delicious meal plans and shopping lists to make your life easier. We recommend that you map out your meals and snacks for a full week and make a shopping list from this, taking into consideration what you already have at home. We have shopping lists that correspond to the meal plans, to make this easy for you.

Storecupboard staples

We purposefully made the meal plans with lots of built-in flexibility so that you can pick and choose to suit your palate. As long as the food fits with our food rules, get stuck into it! We have limited the cooking and prep to 3 days to make it sustainable, and it will probably take you 2–3 hours each time to prep the food for the following couple of days. If you are quick it may only take you about an hour at a time, so it really depends on your cooking experience. Storecupboard ingredients are great, as they have a long shelf life and can help flesh out a dinner. Below we'll run through some of our storecupboard staples for a wholefood plant-based kitchen, and label reading to help support you once you're in the grocery store.

Tinned beans and pulses
- [ ] Black beans
- [ ] Butter beans
- [ ] Chickpeas
- [ ] Kidney beans
- [ ] Lentils

Dried pulses
- [ ] Lentils (our favourites are split red lentils and brown/green lentils)
- [ ] Mung dal
- [ ] Yellow or green split peas

Nuts, seeds and dried fruit
NUTS
- [ ] Whole almonds
- [ ] Flaked almonds (nice for garnishing)
- [ ] Cashew nuts
- [ ] Walnuts
- [ ] Pecan nuts (tend to be a bit more expensive)

SEEDS
- [ ] Pumpkin seeds
- [ ] Sesame seeds
- [ ] Sunflower seeds
- [ ] Chia seeds
- [ ] Flax seeds

DRIED FRUIT
- [ ] Apricots (try to buy the brown ones, as they are not dried with sulphur and taste juicier)
- [ ] Goji berries
- [ ] Medjool dates/pitted dates
- [ ] Sun-dried tomatoes

Wholegrains and pasta

- ☐ Short-grain brown rice (our preferred rice choice)
- ☐ Brown basmati rice
- ☐ Wholemeal couscous
- ☐ Quinoa (it's higher in protein than the average grain)
- ☐ Packs of pre-cooked brown rice/ quinoa (for quick easy dinners)
- ☐ Wholewheat penne/fusilli, etc.
- ☐ Wholewheat noodles
- ☐ Wholewheat spaghetti
- ☐ Gluten-free options: brown rice, buckwheat and lentil pasta or noodles

Condiments

- ☐ Apple cider vinegar
- ☐ Balsamic vinegar
- ☐ Nutritional yeast (you may only get this in a health food store)
- ☐ Tahini
- ☐ Tamari or soy sauce

Fridge bits

- ☐ Kimchi
- ☐ Miso paste
- ☐ Olives (we love black Kalamata olives!)
- ☐ Oat milk or plant milk of choice (see page 102 for more on this)
- ☐ Sauerkraut

Spices and seasonings

- ☐ Salt (fine and coarse are useful to have)
- ☐ Ground black pepper
- ☐ Chilli powder (medium)
- ☐ Chilli flakes
- ☐ Ground cinnamon
- ☐ Ground coriander
- ☐ Coriander seeds
- ☐ Ground cumin
- ☐ Cumin seeds
- ☐ Curry powder (medium)
- ☐ Ground ginger
- ☐ Ground paprika
- ☐ Smoked paprika
- ☐ Ground turmeric

Label reading

Label reading is a really important skill to develop, as it will give you the tools to understand what is in packaged foods and which are healthy choices versus unhealthy ones. We highly recommend that you develop this skill, as making healthy choices without it is very difficult.

LABEL READING RULES

1. **Never believe what is written on the front of a packet.** This is for selling the product, not for ensuring you eat as healthily as possible.
2. **Always read the ingredients list** and the nutritional information on the back of the product – this must be accurate by law.
3. **Ingredients are listed in descending order** according to weight, which means there is the most of the first ingredient in the list and the least of the last ingredient.

FAT

As we discussed earlier on, when buying packaged goods ensure that the fat content is below 10% or close to it and that it ideally doesn't contain any oils. Fat will be listed in weight per the size of the product and per 100g. Simply look at the fat content per 100g and this will give you the amount of fat as a percentage.

SUGAR

If you are concerned about avoiding sugars, make sure there are none in the first few ingredients on the list. Sugar comes in a lot of different forms, though, so lots of food companies cleverly disguise how much sugar is in their products by using multiple different types of sugars – this way 'sugar' is not listed at the top as one of the primary ingredients – sneaky, eh! Other tricks food manufacturers use to hide sugar are using evaporated cane juice and dehydrated honey. By taking out the water these sugars weigh far less, so they go down to the end of the list, but the calorie count is still the same.

We are often asked what is the healthiest sweetener and the reality is none – sweeteners are refined, and ideally we eat as little of them as possible.

Look out for these names in your ingredients list: unrefined sugar cane, fructose, maple syrup, barley malt, sucrose, dextrose, maltose, corn syrup, malt flavouring, high fructose corn syrup, evaporated cane juice, brown sugar, molasses, beet sugar.

REFINED CARBOHYDRATES

Unless a grain has the word 'whole' in front of it, it is very likely a refined carbohydrate. There is another helpful way to identify this: check the fibre content per 100g. Ideally there should be at least 3g of fibre per 100g – if so this is a good indicator that it is a wholegrain.

For example, the following are NOT wholegrains:

- Semolina
- Durum
- Durum wheat
- Enriched durum wheat
- Bleached flour
- Unbleached flour
- Wheat flour
- Enriched wheat flour
- Unbleached enriched wheat flour

By comparison, the following ARE wholegrains:

- Rye flour
- Wholewheat flour
- Whole spelt flour
- Wholemeal couscous

SODIUM/SALT

80–90% of people's salt intake comes from packaged refined foods, so cutting these out dramatically reduces your salt intake. Salt density is how much salt you take compared to how many calories you consume. So if you eat 2,000 calories per day and your salt intake is 2,000mg per day, your salt density is 1mg. We never want our salt density to exceed 1. On average a healthy person in the West eats about 2,200 calories per day. Based on this they should be consuming 2,200mg of salt, at most. So, when it comes to the number of milligrams of salt in a product, it should never be more than the number of calories you eat in a day.

Alternatives

MILK

When it comes to milk, you have a wide variety of choices. All plant-based milks are primarily made up of water and are usually less than 1% fat. Oat milk is our personal favourite. Its natural sweetness means that it goes great in porridge or on cereal, and it's our favourite in coffee too.

Other types include soya milk, almond milk, coconut milk and hazelnut milk. There seem to be more and more varieties of non-dairy milk on the market each year, including quinoa, spelt, rice and hemp.

For coffee drinkers who are used to a frothy cappuccino or latte, oat milk works well, as does rice-almond milk. There are lots of 'made for barista' plant milks that are designed to froth as well as cows' milk. Try out different types and find which one you like the best.

EGGS

For baking there are some great alternatives to eggs that work just as well.

- Flax egg – finely ground flax seeds work well as a binder. The basic ratio is 1 tablespoon of ground flax seeds to 3 tablespoons of water. Stir, then leave it to sit for 3–5 minutes.
- Banana – a banana brings moisture and binds cakes and muffins. Depending on the recipe, use half to a whole banana to replace 1 egg.
- Chia seeds – soaking chia seeds in water gives them a gloopy consistency that can help to bind a mixture in the same way as an egg. A basic ratio is 3 tablespoons of water to 1 tablespoon of ground chia seeds. Stir, then leave to sit for 3–5 minutes.
- Aqua faba or chickpea water (from a tin of chickpeas) can be frothed to mimic egg whites and create egg-less meringues.

There is no real vegan alternative to a fried egg; however, we do have options for vegan 'scrambled eggs' (see page 138) in the breakfast section.

CHEESE

While there are many dairy-free cheeses now available in supermarkets and health food stores, these are often primarily made with coconut oil/nuts and starches and are high in fat. In most cases we avoid these high-fat alternatives (dairy cheese is also very high in saturated fat), but we have a few replacements for you to try:

- Cheese sauce – cashew nuts can be blended with water, nutritional yeast and seasoning to make a great cheese sauce. See the creamy red pepper pasta on page 234 and the no oil carbonara on page 237.
- Parmesan – a great alternative to Parmesan for your pasta is nutritional yeast. While it won't give you the same fat hit, this deactivated yeast has a cheesy flavour and is a great addition to pasta, stews and even popcorn!

BUTTER

There are many dairy-free spreads now available in supermarkets and health food stores, but they're highly processed and do not fit within a wholefood plant-based diet. We recommend using a spread of avocado or hummus on your bread if you're looking to add a bit of fat.

LOW-FODMAP MISO STOCK

Garlic- and onion-free veg stock is usually very hard to come by, so to make an easy Happy Gut veg stock that is low-FODMAP (no onion and garlic), simply add 4 tablespoons of gluten-free miso paste (e.g. brown rice miso) to 2 litres of warm water and mix it through.

Meal plans and shopping lists

We have provided meal plans with corresponding shopping lists to make it as easy as possible for you to start. These are there to help empower you and make starting as easy as possible, but feel free to mix and match our recipes – all the recipes with the heart, shape and skin icons are 'eat as much as you like', as they are high in fibre and low in calories. The even better news is that the food is delicious and will leave you looking for more – which you can have too! The Happy Gut meal plan on page 118 is a FODMAP-controlled approach so is not all-you-can-eat and is specific to the portion size of each recipe.

In terms of our food habits, each of us is starting from a different place: you may be wondering whether you will just be eating salad for 4 weeks or you may be well on your way to a wholefood plant-based diet already. Either way, rest assured that the food is absolutely delicious. For breakfast you could have porridge or toasties, chia seed pudding, scrambled 'eggs' on toast or shakshuka, to name a few. Lunch might be a Lebanese lemon parsley and bean salad or a sweet potato and chickpea soup or even some vegan hoisin duck pancakes. Dinner might be a spicy peanut African stew or creamy spiced black bean quesadillas or even some oil-free lasagna.

We purposefully made the meal plans with lots of built-in flexibility, so that you can pick and choose to suit your palate and your lifestyle and the number of people you are cooking for. All these meal plans are for 4 people, so freeze any leftovers* or eat them the next day. All the meals can be refrigerated and will keep for 3 days in an airtight container.

We have limited the cooking and prep to 3 days to make it sustainable, and these will probably take you approx. 2 hours' prep time to cook the food for the following couple of days. If you are quick it may take you less time – this will depend on your kitchen and cooking experience as well as your enthusiasm! Feel free to add bread and spreads to the lunches too.

* Freezing tip: you can freeze leftovers. Frozen food should be covered and defrosted overnight in the fridge in a suitable container. Defrosted food should not be refrozen unless first cooked to over 70°C for at least 2 minutes before freezing again.

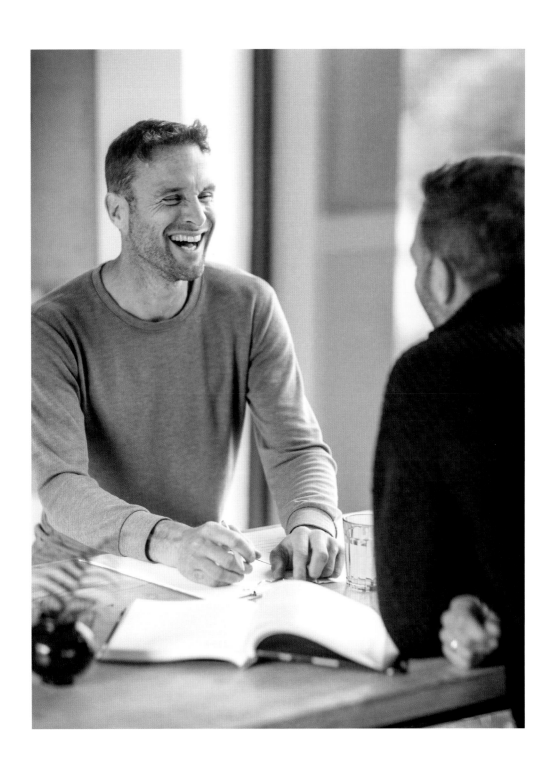

The Happy Heart Serves 4 people

	Monday	Tuesday
Cooking / Prep	• Carrot cake chia pudding • Thai noodle soup • Katsu curry	
Breakfast	Carrot cake chia pudding	Carrot cake chia pudding
Lunch	Thai noodle soup	Thai noodle soup
Dinner	Katsu curry	Katsu curry
Dessert	Fresh fruit (apples, bananas, pears, oranges – whatever your preference), dried fruit of choice, or even try chopped fruit and one of the healthier dessert sauces, or one of the 2 energy ball recipes. Please don't limit yourself to our recipes – once it fits the food rules, go for it!	
Snacks	Fresh fruit (apples, bananas, pears, oranges – whatever your preference), toasties, energy balls, kale crisps, crackers and hummus. Even try chopped fruit and one of the healthier dessert sauces. Please don't limit yourself to our recipes – once it fits the food rules, go for it!	

All our Happy Heart recipes and meal plans are indicated by ♡. In terms of specific recipes, for optimum results we recommend you only eat coconut yoghurt and tinned coconut milk twice a week, and the same goes for our spanakopita recipe on page 248, as these are all slightly higher in fat.

	Wednesday	Thursday	Friday	Saturday / Sunday
	• Vegan shakshuka • Tahini, banana and cinnamon toastie • Vegan Caesar salad • Burrito bowl • Tuscan vegan sausage and bean stew • Easy creamy roasted red pepper pasta			• Matcha and buckwheat almond pancakes • Sweet potato fritters • Easy Mexican enchiladas
	Vegan shakshuka	Tahini, banana and cinnamon toastie	Vegan shakshuka	Matcha and buckwheat almond pancakes
	Vegan Caesar salad	Burrito bowl	Vegan Caesar salad	Sweet potato fritters
	Tuscan vegan sausage and bean stew	Easy creamy roasted red pepper pasta	Tuscan vegan sausage and bean stew	Easy Mexican enchiladas

The Happy Heart

- ☐ fresh ginger
- ☐ avocados
- ☐ beetroot
- ☐ lime
- ☐ courgette
- ☐ white onion
- ☐ red onion
- ☐ red pepper
- ☐ wholemeal bread
- ☐ small ripe tomato
- ☐ small sprig of fresh rosemary
- ☐ tamarind pulp
- ☐ a baguette or other bread
- ☐ medium potatoes
- ☐ cucumber
- ☐ green beans
- ☐ sauerkraut (ideally red, if you can find it)
- ☐ tomato purée
- ☐ non-dairy milk
- ☐ red wine
- ☐ fresh coriander (or other fresh herb)
- ☐ carrots
- ☐ sweet potatoes
- ☐ split red lentils
- ☐ dried Puy/green/brown lentils

- ☐ frozen peas
- ☐ pitted dates
- ☐ fresh coriander
- ☐ oat milk
- ☐ bananas
- ☐ lemons
- ☐ almond butter
- ☐ black sulphur salt or kala namak (or sea salt if you can't get this)
- ☐ baby spinach
- ☐ cashew nuts
- ☐ coconut yoghurt or soy yoghurt
- ☐ mushrooms of choice
- ☐ coconut yoghurt (fat content approx. 10%)
- ☐ kombu/dulse seaweed (optional)
- ☐ oats
- ☐ oyster mushrooms
- ☐ tins of cooked Puy lentils, or other green or brown lentils
- ☐ onion powder
- ☐ fresh red chillies
- ☐ rice flour
- ☐ tins of chopped tomatoes
- ☐ firm tofu
- ☐ silken tofu

- [ ] raisins
- [ ] sesame seeds
- [ ] sun-dried tomatoes
- [ ] flaked almonds
- [ ] tomatoes
- [ ] bay leaves
- [ ] cherry tomatoes
- [ ] leeks
- [ ] lettuce
- [ ] chilli flakes
- [ ] apple cider vinegar
- [ ] balsamic vinegar
- [ ] black or yellow mustard seeds
- [ ] fresh thyme
- [ ] chia seeds
- [ ] cumin seeds
- [ ] curry powder
- [ ] garlic
- [ ] garlic powder
- [ ] gherkins
- [ ] gluten-free burger buns
- [ ] ground allspice
- [ ] ground cinnamon
- [ ] ground flax seeds
- [ ] ground turmeric
- [ ] smoked paprika
- [ ] maple syrup
- [ ] mirin (optional)
- [ ] mustard
- [ ] nutritional yeast
- [ ] quinoa

- [ ] sesame seeds
- [ ] sunflower oil
- [ ] tamari/soy sauce
- [ ] vanilla extract
- [ ] veg stock
- [ ] wholemeal bread
- [ ] wholemeal couscous/ brown rice/quinoa
- [ ] tin of chickpeas
- [ ] walnuts
- [ ] raisins
- [ ] cocoa powder

The Happy Skin Serves 4 people

	Monday	Tuesday
Cooking / Prep	• Banoffee overnight oats • Maple roasted root veg soup • No oil creamy lasagna	
Breakfast	Banoffee overnight oats	Banoffee overnight oats
Lunch	Maple roasted root veg soup	Maple roasted root veg soup
Dinner	No oil creamy lasagna	No oil creamy lasagna
Dessert	Fresh fruit (apples, bananas, pears, orange – whatever your preference), dried fruit of choice, or even try chopped fruit and one of the healthier dessert sauces, or one of the 2 energy ball recipes. Please don't limit yourself to our recipes – once it fits the food rules, go for it!	
Snacks	Fresh fruit (apples, bananas, pears, orange – whatever your preference), toasties, energy balls, kale crisps, crackers and hummus. Even try chopped fruit and one of the healthier dessert sauces. Please don't limit yourself to our recipes – once it fits the food rules, go for it!	

All our Happy Skin recipes and meal plans are indicated by 🖐. These recipes have no calorie-counting or quantity restriction, so eat as much as you want. These recipes are high in antioxidants to protect your skin, fibre that will feed your healthy gut bacteria, water to keep your skin fresh and hydrated and, most importantly, they taste fantastic.

	Wednesday	Thursday	Friday	Saturday / Sunday
	• Carrot cake chia pudding • Avocado, tomato and garlic toastie • Japanese teriyaki tofu and grain bowl • Grilled veggie and tofu kebabs with chimichurri sauce • Quick burger • Humble lentil stew with raita			• Scrambled 'eggs' on toast • Lentil sambar soup • Cottage pie with sweet potato mash and coriander drizzle
	Carrot cake chia pudding	Avocado, tomato and garlic toastie	Carrot cake chia pudding	Scrambled 'eggs' on toast
	Japanese teriyaki tofu and grain bowl	Grilled veggie and tofu kebabs with chimichurri sauce	Japanese teriyaki tofu and grain bowl	Lentil sambar soup
	Quick burger	Humble lentil stew with raita	Quick burger	Cottage pie with sweet potato mash and coriander drizzle

The Happy Skin

- [ ] maple syrup
- [ ] banana
- [ ] spring onions/scallions
- [ ] fresh green chilli
- [ ] leek
- [ ] lemon
- [ ] lemongrass stalk
- [ ] almond butter
- [ ] gram flour or gluten-free flour
- [ ] block of firm tofu
- [ ] tins of sweetcorn
- [ ] jars of roasted red peppers in brine
- [ ] tin of coconut milk
- [ ] yellow pepper
- [ ] cucumber
- [ ] cherry tomatoes
- [ ] matcha powder
- [ ] buckwheat flour
- [ ] gluten-free oats
- [ ] gram flour
- [ ] kale
- [ ] oyster mushrooms
- [ ] non-dairy milk
- [ ] soy yoghurt/vegan mayo
- [ ] strawberries
- [ ] sunflower oil

- [ ] tempeh
- [ ] fresh flat-leaf parsley
- [ ] ground almonds
- [ ] sweet potatoes
- [ ] carrots
- [ ] stalks of celery
- [ ] vanilla extract
- [ ] tins of black beans
- [ ] tins of chickpeas
- [ ] tins of butter beans
- [ ] yellow peppers
- [ ] cashew nuts
- [ ] frozen peas
- [ ] wholemeal couscous
- [ ] tomato purée
- [ ] fresh basil
- [ ] almond milk
- [ ] avocados
- [ ] baby gem lettuces
- [ ] limes
- [ ] onions
- [ ] red peppers
- [ ] wholemeal burrito wraps
- [ ] firm tofu
- [ ] vegan sausages
- [ ] wholewheat or brown rice noodles

- [ ] brown basmati or short-grain brown rice
- [ ] bay leaves
- [ ] cherry tomatoes
- [ ] fresh red chillies
- [ ] tins of chopped tomatoes
- [ ] potatoes
- [ ] red onions
- [ ] mushrooms
- [ ] oat milk
- [ ] capers
- [ ] green beans
- [ ] medium wholemeal/corn tortillas
- [ ] sprigs of fresh thyme
- [ ] brown breadcrumbs
- [ ] fresh ginger
- [ ] apple cider vinegar
- [ ] black sulphur salt or kala namak (or sea salt if you can't get this)
- [ ] cayenne pepper
- [ ] chilli powder
- [ ] cocoa powder
- [ ] coconut sugar or brown sugar
- [ ] cumin seeds
- [ ] curry powder
- [ ] dried thyme
- [ ] flour
- [ ] garam masala
- [ ] garlic
- [ ] garlic powder
- [ ] fresh coriander

- [ ] ground allspice
- [ ] ground cinnamon
- [ ] ground coriander
- [ ] ground cumin
- [ ] ground flax seed
- [ ] ground turmeric
- [ ] light tahini
- [ ] onion powder
- [ ] smoked paprika
- [ ] tamari/soy sauce
- [ ] tomato purée
- [ ] veg stock
- [ ] vinegar
- [ ] wholemeal bread
- [ ] walnuts
- [ ] raisins
- [ ] cocoa powder

The Happy Shape Serves 4 people

	Monday	Tuesday
Cooking / Prep	• Scrambled 'eggs' on toast • Polish potato cakes with cannellini beans • Spicy African peanut stew	
Breakfast	Scrambled 'eggs' on toast	Scrambled 'eggs' on toast
Lunch	Polish potato cakes with cannellini beans	Polish potato cakes with cannellini beans
Dinner	Spicy African peanut stew	Spicy African peanut stew
Dessert	Fresh fruit (apples, bananas, pears, oranges – whatever your preference), dried fruit of choice, or even try chopped fruit and one of the healthier dessert sauces, or one of the 2 energy ball recipes. Please don't limit yourself to our recipes – once it fits the food rules, go for it!	
Snacks	Fresh fruit (apples, bananas, pears, oranges – whatever your preference), toasties, energy balls, kale crisps, crackers and hummus. Even try chopped fruit and one of the healthier dessert sauces. Please don't limit yourself to our recipes – once it fits the food rules, go for it!	

All our Happy Shape recipes and meal plans are indicated by ◯. Happy Shape is an all-you-can-eat philosophy, no need for calorie-counting or portion control. All our recipes are low to medium energy density, so are naturally low in calories and fat, while at the same time being high in water and fibre, so they're great at filling you up.

	Wednesday	Thursday	Friday	Saturday / Sunday
	• 3-grain coconut porridge • Carrot cake chia pudding • Eat your greens soup • Peanut satay tofu pot • Spaghetti bolognese • Japanese veg and noodle ramen			• Banoffee overnight oats • Grilled veggie and tofu kebabs with Chimichurri sauce • Greek spanakopita with sweet potato
	3-grain coconut porridge	Carrot cake chia pudding	3-grain coconut porridge	Banoffee overnight oats
	Eat your greens soup	Peanut satay tofu pot	Eat your greens soup	Grilled veggie and tofu kebabs with chimichurri sauce
	Spaghetti bolognese	Japanese veg and noodle ramen	Spaghetti bolognese	Greek spanakopita with sweet potato

The Happy Shape

- [ ] bay leaf
- [ ] courgette
- [ ] red onion
- [ ] red pepper
- [ ] shallot
- [ ] fresh ginger
- [ ] beansprouts
- [ ] tin of cannellini beans
- [ ] tin of chickpeas
- [ ] celeriac
- [ ] a baguette or other bread
- [ ] white cabbage
- [ ] oyster mushrooms
- [ ] pot barley
- [ ] red or white quinoa
- [ ] fresh coriander or parsley
- [ ] coconut yoghurt
- [ ] peanut butter
- [ ] cashew nuts
- [ ] pitted dates
- [ ] fresh chives
- [ ] fresh dill
- [ ] fresh mint
- [ ] tinned cooked lentils
- [ ] red wine
- [ ] bananas

- [ ] lemons
- [ ] vegan puff pastry
- [ ] spring onions/scallions
- [ ] sweet potatoes
- [ ] almond butter
- [ ] tins of chopped tomatoes
- [ ] black sulphur salt or kala namak (or sea salt if you can't get this)
- [ ] baby spinach
- [ ] cherry tomatoes
- [ ] coconut yoghurt (fat content approx. 10%)
- [ ] oats
- [ ] fresh flat-leaf parsley
- [ ] carrots
- [ ] fresh red chillies
- [ ] onions
- [ ] gram flour or buckwheat flour
- [ ] leeks
- [ ] limes
- [ ] nests of brown rice noodles
- [ ] peanut butter
- [ ] toasted peanuts
- [ ] frozen spinach
- [ ] gluten-free spaghetti (brown rice is our favourite)

- [ ] silken tofu (or firm tofu if you can't get silken tofu)
- [ ] sweet potatoes
- [ ] tomatoes
- [ ] raisins
- [ ] sunflower oil
- [ ] firm tofu
- [ ] flaked almonds
- [ ] rolled oats
- [ ] oat milk
- [ ] tin of coconut milk
- [ ] potatoes
- [ ] cherry tomatoes
- [ ] fresh basil
- [ ] apple cider vinegar
- [ ] chia seeds
- [ ] chilli flakes
- [ ] fresh or dried oregano
- [ ] garlic
- [ ] garlic powder
- [ ] grated nutmeg
- [ ] ground allspice
- [ ] ground cinnamon
- [ ] ground coriander
- [ ] ground cumin
- [ ] ground turmeric
- [ ] ground flax seeds
- [ ] sweet paprika
- [ ] non-dairy milk
- [ ] nutritional yeast
- [ ] onion powder

- [ ] quinoa
- [ ] red or white wine vinegar
- [ ] sauerkraut
- [ ] sesame seeds
- [ ] vanilla extract
- [ ] veg stock
- [ ] wholemeal bread
- [ ] walnuts
- [ ] raisins
- [ ] cocoa powder

The Happy Gut Serves 4 people

	Monday	Tuesday
Cooking / Prep	• Happy Gut 5-minute berry chia jam • Gluten-free porridge bread • Maple roasted root veg soup • Low-FODMAP Malaysian laksa curry	
Breakfast	Happy Gut 5-minute berry chia jam Gluten-free porridge bread	Happy Gut 5-minute berry chia jam Gluten-free porridge bread
Lunch	Maple roasted root veg soup	Maple roasted root veg soup
Dinner	Low-FODMAP Malaysian laksa curry	Low-FODMAP Malaysian laksa curry
Snacks	Maple and seed flapjacks	Maple and seed flapjacks

All our Happy Gut recipes and meal plans are indicated by ⊜. The Happy Gut recipes are low-FODMAP, which is quite technical and very specific around quantities. The Happy Gut course is not an all-you-can-eat approach like our other 3 plans because of the controlled FODMAP approach. Please follow the recipes and specific quantities.

	Wednesday	Thursday	Friday	Saturday / Sunday
	• Easy strawberry muffin • Quick easy porridge • Happy Gut high protein quinoa salad • Lentil sambar soup • Japanese veg and noodle ramen • Spinach and butter bean curry			• Light crunchy granola • Happy Gut toasted wholemeal pitta with hummus, rocket and tomato • Quick burger
	Easy strawberry muffin	Quick easy porridge	Easy strawberry muffin	Light crunchy granola
	Happy Gut high protein quinoa salad	Lentil sambar soup	Vegan Caesar salad	Sweet potato fritters
	Japanese veg and noodle ramen	Spinach and butter bean curry	Japanese veg and noodle ramen	Quick burger
	Kale crisps	Maple and seed flapjacks	Low-FODMAP hummus and rice cakes	Maple and seed flapjacks

The Happy Gut

- ☐ ground flax seed
- ☐ wholemeal pitta breads
- ☐ lemons
- ☐ beansprouts
- ☐ courgette
- ☐ ripe tomato
- ☐ green beans
- ☐ pecan nuts/walnuts
- ☐ cranberry juice
- ☐ freeze-dried strawberries
- ☐ fresh chives
- ☐ fresh coriander (or other fresh herb)
- ☐ fresh mint
- ☐ bay leaves
- ☐ flaked almonds
- ☐ split red lentils
- ☐ tin of butter beans
- ☐ ground almonds
- ☐ cherry tomatoes
- ☐ broccoli florets
- ☐ spring onions/scallions
- ☐ baby spinach or similar greens
- ☐ oyster mushrooms
- ☐ tofu/tempeh
- ☐ coconut milk

- ☐ full-fat coconut milk
- ☐ rice or almond milk
- ☐ tins of chopped tomatoes
- ☐ strawberries
- ☐ goji berries
- ☐ raisins
- ☐ fresh red chillies
- ☐ coconut yoghurt
- ☐ blueberries
- ☐ limes
- ☐ desiccated coconut
- ☐ potatoes
- ☐ sprigs of fresh thyme
- ☐ frozen edamame beans/ frozen peas
- ☐ raspberries
- ☐ leeks
- ☐ fresh ginger
- ☐ carrots
- ☐ nests of brown rice noodles
- ☐ gluten-free flour or buckwheat flour
- ☐ mixed salad leaves
- ☐ rocket
- ☐ kale
- ☐ tin of chickpeas

- [ ] apple cider vinegar
- [ ] baking powder
- [ ] balsamic vinegar
- [ ] bicarbonate of soda
- [ ] black or yellow mustard seeds
- [ ] chia seeds
- [ ] coriander seeds
- [ ] cumin seeds
- [ ] curry powder
- [ ] fresh coriander/basil
- [ ] gluten-free burger buns
- [ ] gluten-free oats
- [ ] ground cumin
- [ ] ground flax seeds
- [ ] ground turmeric
- [ ] maple syrup
- [ ] mixed seeds
- [ ] nutritional yeast
- [ ] rice flour
- [ ] quinoa
- [ ] sauerkraut
- [ ] sesame seeds
- [ ] sunflower seeds
- [ ] pumpkin seeds
- [ ] sunflower oil
- [ ] tamari
- [ ] tamarind pulp
- [ ] vanilla extract
- [ ] veg stock (garlic- and onion-free)
- [ ] cayenne pepper

Make your own

	Monday	Tuesday
Cooking / Prep		
Breakfast		
Lunch		
Dinner		
Dessert		
Snacks		

	Wednesday	Thursday	Friday	Saturday / Sunday

REC

PES

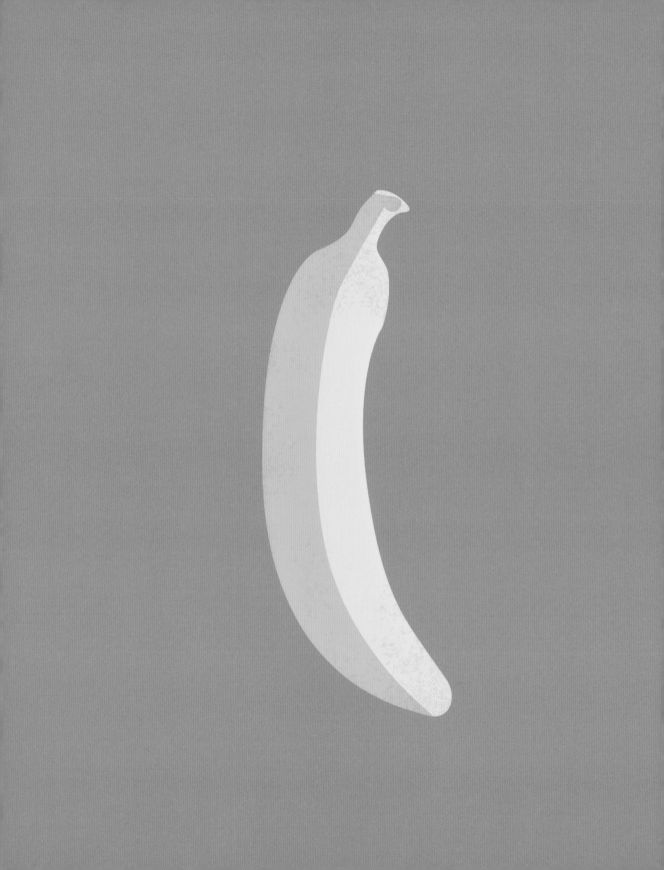

Chapter 8

Breakfast

From shakshuka, to banoffee overnight oats, to matcha and buckwheat almond pancakes, this section will satisfy your quick, healthy mid-week breakfast desires as well as your more elaborate weekend brunches.

Banoffee Overnight Oats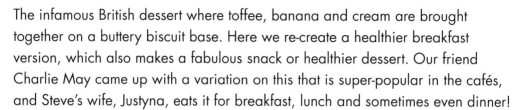

The infamous British dessert where toffee, banana and cream are brought together on a buttery biscuit base. Here we re-create a healthier breakfast version, which also makes a fabulous snack or healthier dessert. Our friend Charlie May came up with a variation on this that is super-popular in the cafés, and Steve's wife, Justyna, eats it for breakfast, lunch and sometimes even dinner!

Serves 4
Takes 10 minutes (plus soaking time)

2 bananas
200g coconut yoghurt (fat content approx. 10%)

Date caramel
150g pitted dates
2 tablespoons almond butter
½ teaspoon vanilla extract
a pinch of salt

Bircher muesli
250g oats
40g raisins
20g chia seeds
600ml oat milk
a pinch of ground cinnamon

Caramelized almond sprinkle
50g flaked almonds
2 tablespoons maple syrup

Fill and boil the kettle. Cover the pitted dates with 250ml of boiling water and leave to soak for 5 minutes.

Mix all the ingredients for the bircher muesli together and leave to soak for at least 30 minutes, or overnight, if possible.

To make the caramelized almonds, heat a non-stick pan on a medium heat. When it's hot, add the almonds and cook for 4–6 minutes, until they start to turn golden, making sure to stir regularly to avoid them burning. Once they are golden, remove the pan from the heat. Add the maple syrup and stir quickly to make sure you coat each nut. Continue to stir for a minute, until the maple syrup has started to harden.

Drain the dates and put them into a food processor. Add another 100ml of boiling water, the almond butter, vanilla and a pinch of salt, and blend until it reaches a smooth caramel-like texture.

Peel the bananas and slice them into thin coin shapes.

We like to serve this in clear glasses so that we can see the layers. Put a layer of caramel at the bottom of each glass (divide the amount between four glasses). Next divide up the bircher muesli, followed by a serving of banana – it looks great if you put the bananas facing out around the glass on the inside, so you can really see it's a banoffee. Add a generous dollop of coconut yoghurt and top with some caramelized almonds. Enjoy!

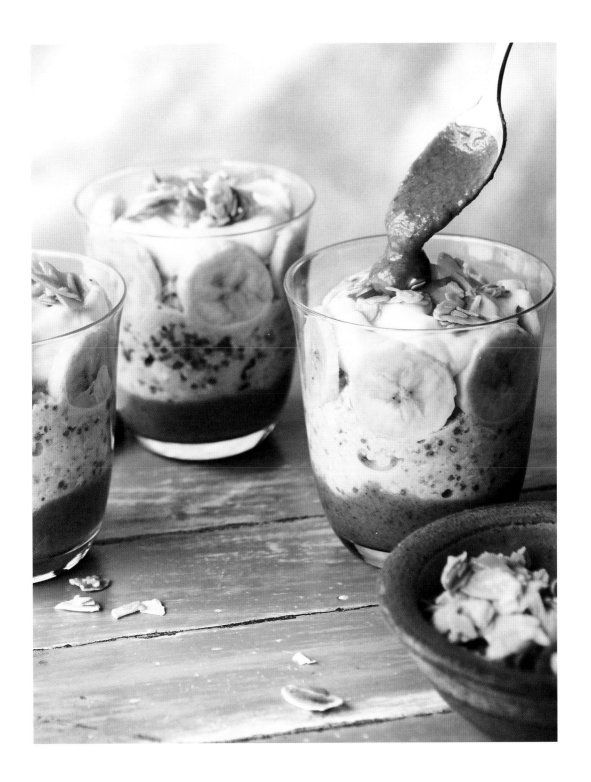

Carrot Cake Chia Pudding

Carrot cake has always been one of Steve's favourites, so he decided to extend his love for it and see if he could come up with a way to enjoy a healthier version for brekkie – this was born out of that idea and it really works!

Serves 4

Takes 10 minutes (plus soaking time)

Chia pudding

30g walnuts
30g carrots
40g chia seeds
300ml almond milk
(or rice milk)
30g raisins
2 tablespoons cocoa powder
30ml maple syrup
a pinch of ground cinnamon
a pinch of ground allspice

To serve

300g coconut yoghurt
(find one with under
15% fat content)

Roughly chop the walnuts and grate the carrots.

In a large bowl, mix together all the ingredients for the chia pudding (leaving 1 tablespoon of walnuts and a little of the grated carrot aside to garnish). Leave to soak for 30 minutes or overnight in the fridge and give it a good stir before serving.

Divide half the chia pudding between four jars or glasses, followed by half the coconut yoghurt. Add the rest of the chia pudding next, and finally another layer of yoghurt. Sprinkle with the reserved chopped walnuts and grated carrot and serve.

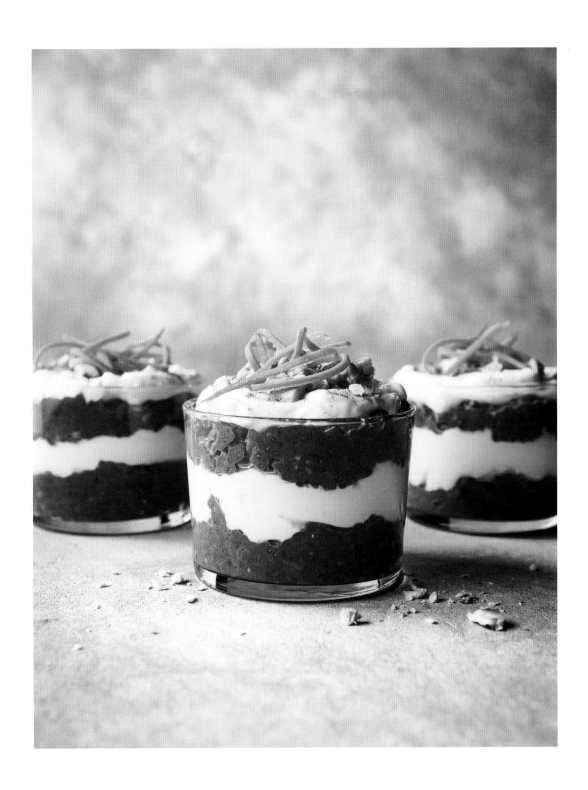

Porridge 3 Ways

Oat Groats ♡ ⊛ ⊘

This is possibly the healthiest way to consume oats, due to the higher fibre and more wholegrain nature. Once soaked overnight they have almost a short-grain brown rice feel, and when soaked in rice milk they become sweet and lovely.

Serves 2 (2 x 240g servings)
Takes 25 minutes (plus soaking time)

120g oat groats
180ml rice milk
180ml water
a pinch of salt

Put all the ingredients into a pan and leave to soak, ideally overnight – but if you forget, that's OK.

Bring to the boil, then reduce to a simmer for 25 minutes.

See box opposite for some topping suggestions.

Quick Easy Porridge ♡ ⊛ ⊘ ⊜

We tend to eat porridge 360 days a year – sometimes I think it's in our bloodstream! Our friend Paul Buggle once cooked it with half non-dairy milk, half water, and it was the creamiest, most wonderful porridge – since that day we've never looked back!

Makes 1 large bowl for a hungry porridge lover, or serves 2
Takes 10 minutes

100g rolled oats (use gluten-free oats for a Happy Gut-friendly version)
250ml water
270ml non-dairy milk of preference (rice or almond milk are both Happy Gut-friendly)

Put all the ingredients into a pan and bring to the boil, stirring regularly. Once boiling, it's good to go! Add more non-dairy milk if you prefer a looser porridge, or else leave to boil and reduce while stirring if you prefer it thicker. In Ireland we love a thicker style of porridge.

See box opposite for some topping suggestions.

3-grain Coconut Porridge ♡ ✋ ⃠

A nice upgrade in grain varieties here – the quinoa adds a lovely soft bite and earthiness, which the coconut milk balances out beautifully. This is a delicious celebration of porridge.

Serves 2–3
Takes 20 minutes

100g red or white quinoa
50g rolled oats
100g pot barley
100ml coconut milk (from a tin)
750ml water
1 teaspoon vanilla extract

Put all the ingredients into a large pan. Bring to the boil, then reduce to a simmer, leaving the lid slightly ajar, and leave to cook until it thickens up nicely (about 20 minutes).

See box below for some topping suggestions.

Porridge Toppings

Toppings can elevate porridge into something beautiful. The key to a good porridge topping is to hit as many different textures as possible, so try to have something crunchy, fruity, creamy and something unexpected.

Something crunchy	toasted seeds (page 160)	granola (page 136)	1 tablespoon of almond butter	a drizzle of tahini
Something fruity	fruit compote (page 135)	apple sauce (page 273)	fresh berries	seasonal fruit
Something creamy	coconut yoghurt	soy yoghurt	almond yoghurt	cashew yoghurt
Something unexpected	cocoa nibs	dessert sauces (page 272)	a pinch of ground cinnamon	1 teaspoon of maple syrup

Gluten-free Porridge Bread ♡ ⑯ ◌ ⑱

The recipe was born out of our Happy Gut course, where participants were looking for a 100% wholemeal gluten-free loaf. Simple, tasty and hearty, this bread is based on an Irish porridge bread. It goes magic with the chia jam on the opposite page.

Makes 1x approx. 700g loaf
Serves 8
Takes 60 minutes

1 tablespoon ground flax seeds
400g coconut yoghurt
1 tablespoon molasses or maple syrup
300g gluten-free oat flakes
2 teaspoons bicarbonate of soda
4 tablespoons mixed seeds
½ teaspoon salt

Preheat the oven to 170°C fan/190°C.

First, make the flax egg: put the ground flax seeds into a cup and add 3 tablespoons of water. Stir, then leave to sit for 5 minutes.

Put the coconut yoghurt, flax egg and molasses into a mixing bowl and stir well.

Next, mix the oats, bicarbonate of soda, seeds and salt in a separate bowl. Add this to the yoghurt mixture and stir thoroughly. It will be quite a wet batter but will dry out once baked.

Place in a greased or parchment-lined 1lb loaf tin and bake in the preheated oven for 50 minutes. Take out of the oven, remove from the tin and leave to cool fully on a wire rack before slicing.

Fruit Compote ♡ 🖐 ⃠

This goes great on top of porridge, with granola, with pancakes, and you can even use it to sweeten a curry. If you are feeling fancy you could maybe add some star anise and cinnamon sticks. This recipe makes enough for a few days – it will keep for at least a week in your fridge.

Makes 600g
Takes 20 minutes

600g frozen berries
   (strawberries, raspberries,
   blueberries)
2 tablespoons maple syrup
1 teaspoon ground cinnamon
   (optional)

Put the frozen berries into a medium pan along with 4 tablespoons of water and place on a high heat. Bring to the boil, then reduce the heat to a simmer.

Add the maple syrup and the cinnamon (if using), then leave to simmer for 15–20 minutes, or longer if you have time – the longer you leave it, the thicker and sweeter your compote will get (it will thicken as it cools, too).

Happy Gut 5-minute Berry Chia Jam ⊜

This is great spread on gluten-free bread, or even served on top of a bowl of porridge. It also goes well with a chia pudding, with some coconut yoghurt on top. It keeps for a week in the fridge, but you will probably have eaten it before then!

Makes 400–500ml
Serves 10
Takes 10–15 minutes

125g strawberries
60g raspberries
40g blueberries
100ml cranberry juice
100ml maple syrup
5 tablespoons chia seeds

Put all the ingredients into a pan and place it on a high heat. Bring to the boil, then lower to a simmer and allow to reduce for a few minutes, stirring occasionally so it doesn't stick.

The jam is ready when it starts to turn a monotone colour. You can use the back of a wooden spoon to encourage the fruit to break down. If you want a smoother texture, use an immersion/stick blender or a food processor or blender.

Leave to cool and firm up.

Light Crunchy Granola ✋ ☺

This works perfectly as a light snack eaten on the go on its own, served with almond milk as a breakfast, with coconut yoghurt and fruit as a cooling summer brekkie, or on top of piping hot porridge to add crunch and sweetness. Easy to make and really delicious! If you can get some freeze-dried strawberries, they really add colour, subtle undertone and vibrancy to this granola.

*Makes approx. 500g
(10 servings)*
Takes approx. 45 minutes

400g jumbo oats (use gluten-free for a Happy Gut-friendly version)
40ml sunflower oil
60ml date syrup or maple syrup
50g desiccated coconut
a pinch of salt
a pinch of ground cinnamon (optional)
30g goji berries
10g freeze-dried strawberries
30g raisins

Preheat the oven to 160°C fan/180°C.

In a large bowl, mix together all the ingredients, except the dried fruit. Pour on to a baking tray measuring approx. 36cm x 27cm.

Bake in the preheated oven for 30 minutes, stirring the granola twice during that time so that it bakes evenly.

Remove from the oven and leave to cool for 15 minutes. Add the dried fruit (goji berries, raisins and freeze-dried strawberries) and mix well.

Store in an airtight container – it will keep fresh for 6 weeks.

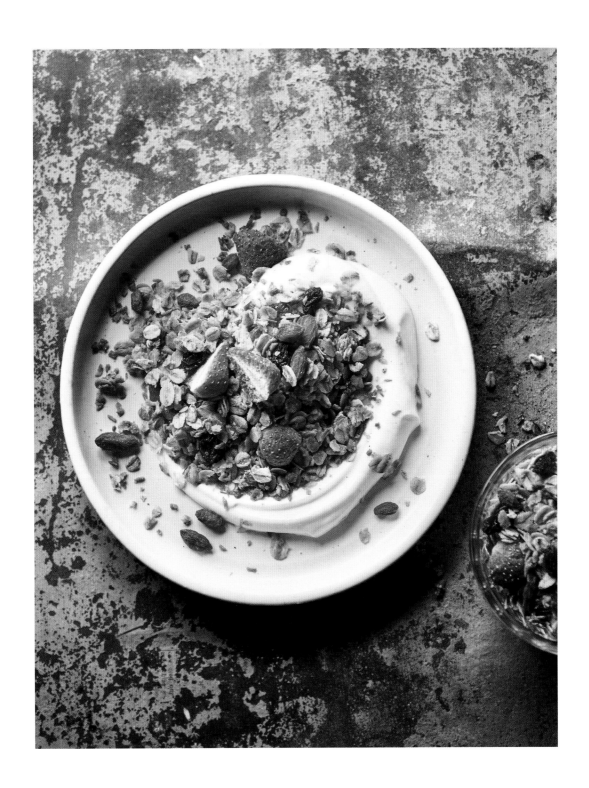

Scrambled 'Eggs' on Toast ♡ ✋ ⦸

Such a simple nourishing breakfast. I remember as a young kid coming back from hospital and us calling in on our granny on the way home. She made us toast cut into strips with scrambled egg and called it egg and soldiers. It felt like the most simple, nourishing but satisfying meal, and even thinking back on it puts a smile on my face. This tofu scramble is delicious, and if you can get the black sulphur salt it really does give an egg-like taste. This one's for you, Granny!

Serves 4
Takes 15 minutes

400g silken tofu (or firm tofu if you can't get this)
3 teaspoons tamari/soy sauce (make sure to use gf soy sauce if you need to avoid gluten)
¾ teaspoon onion powder
½ teaspoon ground turmeric
⅔ teaspoon black sulphur salt or kala namak (or any sea salt if you can't get this)
4 slices of your favourite wholemeal bread
200g cherry tomatoes

Drain the tofu to remove any liquid, then put into a bowl and mash until crumbled. Add the tamari/soy sauce, onion powder and turmeric, and mix well.

Heat a non-stick pan on a medium heat. Once hot, add the mixture and fry, stirring continuously. If it starts to catch, add 1 teaspoon of water to help loosen it from the pan. Cook for 3–4 minutes, until the tofu has started to turn a yellow colour similar to scrambled eggs. Remove from the heat and sprinkle with the black sulphur salt.

Toast your bread to your liking. For the cherry tomatoes, just add them to the hot pan once the tofu is ready and cook for 2–3 minutes until the skins start to wrinkle and they char ever so slightly. Serve together and enjoy!

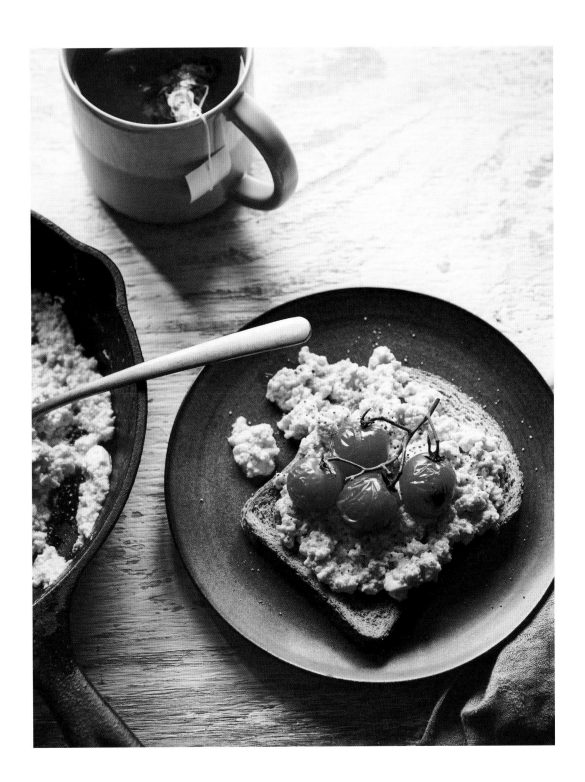

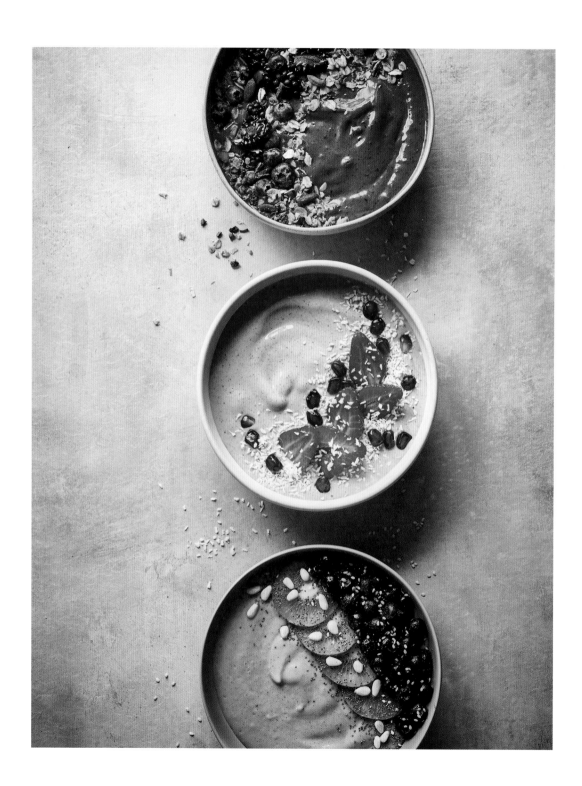

Smoothie Bowls 3 Ways ♡ 🖐 ⊘

Smoothie bowls are a thick blend of wholefoods with almost an ice-cream-like consistency. They are normally eaten with a spoon rather than a straw, meaning you eat slowly rather than gulp, which promotes more mindful eating. Below we give you three of our favourite recipes and a framework to create your own.

	Blueberry and avocado	Choc-oat-late berry bowl	Pomegranate, strawberries and cream
Base (blitz these together in a blender until smooth)	100g frozen blueberries 1 frozen banana (no skin) ½ a Hass avocado a handful of baby spinach (30g) 250ml oat milk or non-dairy milk of choice ½ a lime, juiced 1 tablespoon ground flax seeds	1 frozen banana (no skin) 200g frozen berries 150ml oat milk or non-dairy milk of choice (hazelnut goes great for a Nutella-like note) 4 tablespoons cocoa powder 1 tablespoon tahini 1 tablespoon maple syrup	80g pomegranate seeds 1 frozen banana (no skin) 200g frozen strawberries 150g coconut yoghurt/ soy yoghurt 1 teaspoon vanilla extract
Pick 'n' mix toppings (mix and match your favourite toppings – get curious and try out different combinations)	light crunchy granola (see page 136) goji berries toasted nuts of choice, e.g. flaked almonds, pine nuts, cashews toasted seeds, e.g. sunflower, sesame, pumpkin (see page 160) chia seeds toasted desiccated coconut cocoa nibs pomegranate seeds sliced fruit of choice dried mulberries or sliced dates, dried mango, or even sliced pitted prunes or apricots		

Toastie Spreads

Each of these makes one serving and takes 5–10 minutes.

Avocado, Tomato and Garlic ♡ 👋 ⊘ 🖐

Based on the Catalan dish *pan tomaca*, here we rub the toast with raw garlic to create a simple garlic bread, then add mashed avocado and top with diced seasoned ripe tomatoes for a super-tasty favourite of ours. This makes a wonderful snack, brekkie or lazy dinner.

¼ of an avocado (40g)
a pinch of salt and ground
   black pepper
a squeeze of lemon
   juice (3ml)
1 small ripe tomato (80g)
1 slice of wholemeal bread
a pinch of chilli flakes
   (optional)

Mash the avocado flesh in a bowl with a small pinch of salt and a tiny squeeze of lemon juice until it's nice and smooth. Finely dice the tomato.

Toast your bread and put it on a plate, then spread it with a nice even layer of mashed avocado. Top with diced tomato, a sprinkle of salt and pepper and some chilli flakes if you like it hot.

Tahini, Banana and Cinnamon ♡ 👋 ⊘ 🖐

Our chef mom, Dorene Palmer, used to love smearing a nice lather of tahini followed by some sliced banana on top of toasted sourdough rye bread. This is surprisingly delicious.

1 slice of wholemeal bread
2 teaspoons light tahini
½ a ripe banana
a pinch of ground cinnamon

Toast your bread and put it on a plate. Ensure the tahini is well stirred, as it often separates in the jar, then spread it over the toast. Thinly slice the banana and put it on top of the tahini, and sprinkle a pinch of cinnamon on top if you're a cinnamon fan, or leave out if you dislike it.

Hummus, Miso and Cucumber ♡ ⊛ ◌ ◎

Miso is such a strong umami flavour that it can be overpowering,
but when softened with hummus and cucumber, its sweetness really stands
out. Definitely one of Steve's favourites, and one the kids won't ever
touch, so he knows he can enjoy it in peace!

3 thin slices of cucumber
1 slice of wholemeal bread
3 tablespoons hummus (see
   page 256)
1 teaspoon miso paste

Cut the cucumber slices into matchsticks. Toast your bread and put it on
a plate, then slather a nice dollop of hummus on top. Spread the miso
thinly over the hummus, carefully as it's so strong in flavour, and top with
the matchsticked cucumber.

Smoky Red Pepper Hummus, Sauerkraut, Cucumber ♡ ✋ ⊘

The sweetness of the red pepper balances the smoky flavour here.
Even if you think you don't like sauerkraut, its acidity and crunch add
so much to this and might really challenge those sauerkraut doubters.

1 slice of wholemeal bread
3 tablespoons roasted red
    pepper smoked hummus
    (see page 257)
20g sauerkraut
3 thin slices of cucumber

Toast your bread and put it on a plate. Smear the red pepper hummus
on the toast, put the sauerkraut on top and decorate with the sliced
cucumber.

Sweet Beet Hummus, Peanut Butter and Rocket ♡ ✋ ⊘

Beetroot is the sweetest of all veg, so it goes well with peanut butter,
also known as groundnut butter, to elevate the flavour, bringing you
a really balanced toastie.

1 slice of wholemeal bread
1 tablespoon peanut
    butter (15g)
4 tablespoons sweet beet
    hummus (60g)
    (see page 257)
a handful of rocket

Toast your bread, put it on a plate and spread it with the peanut butter.
Spread the sweet beet hummus on top and finish with the rocket.

Sweet Chocolate Treat ♡ ✋ ⃠

We used to make a more indulgent variation of this in the café, and Steve's kids used to eat way too many of them! Here is a healthier version that still tastes wonderful.

1 slice of wholemeal bread
3 tablespoons chocolate
    sauce (see page 272)
1 tablespoon coconut yoghurt
a sprinkling of freeze-dried
    raspberry powder or
    goji berries

Toast your bread and put it on a plate, then spread it with the chocolate sauce, bringing it right to the edges. Add the coconut yoghurt and decorate with raspberry powder or goji berries. This makes a lovely breakfast or lunch treat, or a nice healthy dessert.

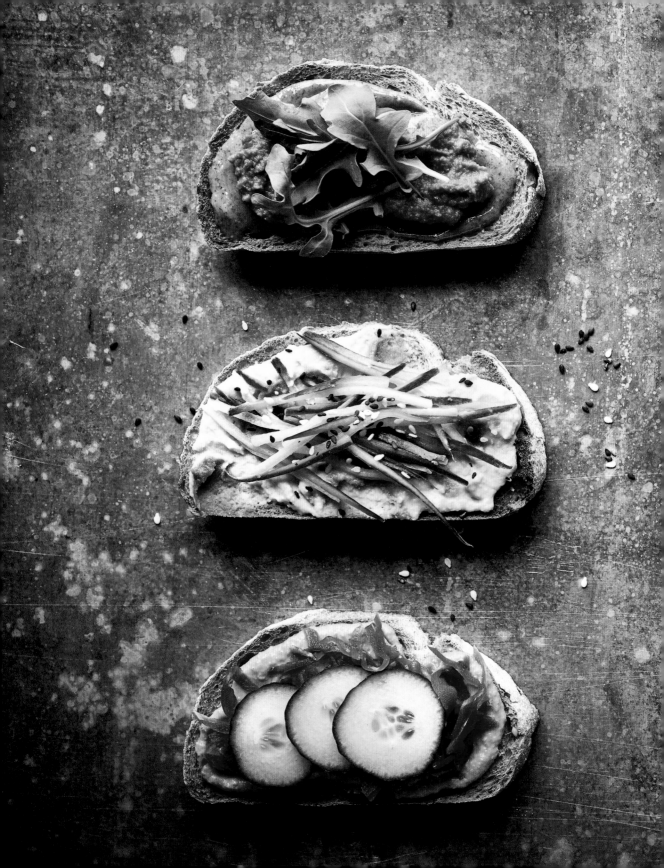

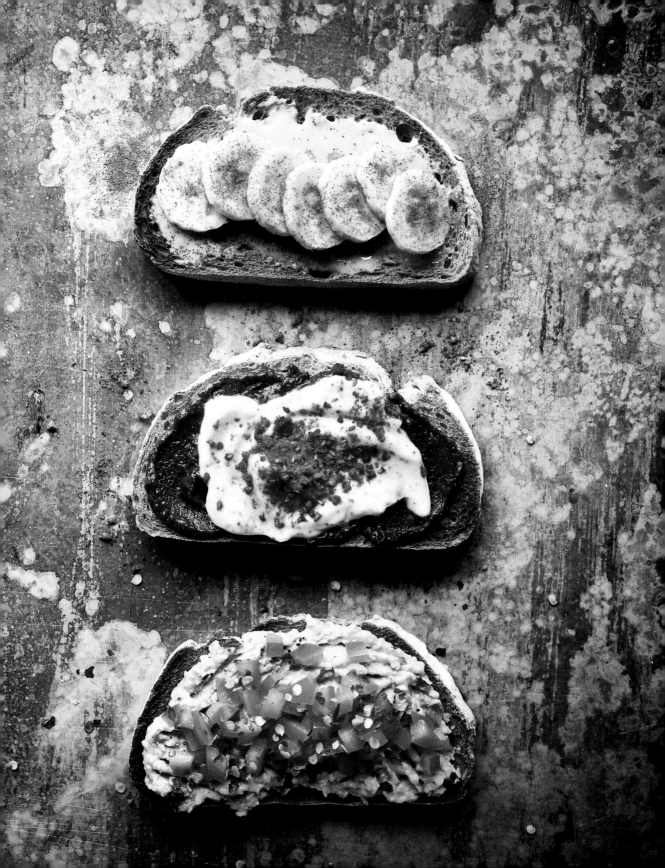

Easy Strawberry Muffins ⊜

Quick, easy and delicious... these have a lovely crispy exterior and will leave you wanting more. They have a wonderful frangipane or bakewell flavour to them.

Makes 8 muffins

Takes 30 minutes

2 tablespoons ground flax seeds

80g gluten-free flour or buckwheat flour

100g gluten-free oats

140g ground almonds

1 teaspoon baking powder

1 teaspoon bicarbonate of soda

150ml sunflower oil

150ml maple syrup

2 teaspoons vanilla extract

125g strawberries (if using frozen, make sure they are thawed)

12g flaked almonds

Preheat the oven to 180°C fan/200°C.

To make your flax eggs, put the ground flax seeds into a bowl, mix with 6 tablespoons of water, and leave to sit while you prepare the rest of the ingredients.

In a large bowl, mix together the dry ingredients: the flour, oats, ground almonds, baking powder and bicarbonate of soda.

Add the sunflower oil to the dry ingredients, along with the maple syrup, vanilla extract and flax eggs, and stir thoroughly until everything is well mixed.

Quarter the strawberries, removing the green tops. Stir three-quarters of the flaked almonds and three-quarters of the strawberries into the batter, keeping the rest to decorate the tops of the muffins later on.

Put eight paper muffin cases into the holes of a muffin tray, and divide the batter equally between them. Decorate the tops of the muffins with the remaining flaked almonds and strawberries, and bake in the preheated oven for about 20 minutes, until they start to turn golden brown on top.

Once cooked, remove from the oven and leave to cool. Serve with some fresh fruit or homemade coconut yoghurt.

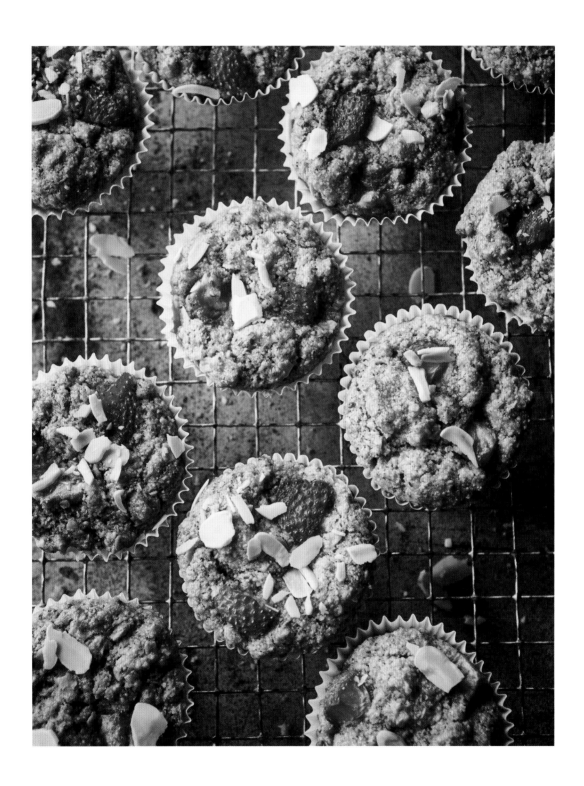

Matcha and Buckwheat Almond Pancakes ♡ ✋ ◌ ⊜

Refined sugar-free and gluten-free, these are also light, fluffy, and go so well when you drizzle over some maple syrup and serve them with berries, coconut yoghurt and almond butter for a yummy brekkie, brunch or treat. Dave makes these at least once a week for his daughters and they love them. Charlie May, a wonderful chef friend who works with us, gave us the inspiration for these.

Makes 4 thin pancakes or 8 fluffy ones (4 servings)
Takes 20 minutes

100g buckwheat flour
25g almond flour or
    almond meal
250ml almond milk
a pinch of salt
2 tablespoons ground
    flax seeds
3 tablespoons maple syrup
1 teaspoon baking powder
½ teaspoon bicarbonate
    of soda
1 tablespoon almond butter
½ tablespoon matcha powder
1 tablespoon oil

To serve
coconut yoghurt
fresh berries
maple syrup

Blend all the ingredients (except the oil) together in a blender or food processor, or simply mix in a bowl until everything is smooth.

Put a non-stick pan on a high heat and give it a few minutes to heat up – you want the pan to be nice and hot. Add 1 tablespoon of oil and move the pan around, spreading the oil to cover most of the surface. Use a sheet of kitchen paper to mop up any extra oil, to minimize calories. You just want the tiniest covering of oil so that your pancakes won't stick to the pan.

Turn the heat down to medium-high and either pour in enough pancake mixture to give a thin coating on the pan, or gently pour in the mixture to make 2 circles. Cook for a few minutes, until bubbles start to form and the top starts to dry out and not look moist anymore.

Using a silicone spatula, turn the pancake, or pancakes, and cook on the other side until a nice golden brown colour. Repeat with the remaining batter until it's all gone.

To serve, pour over some coconut yoghurt and add fresh berries and maple syrup.

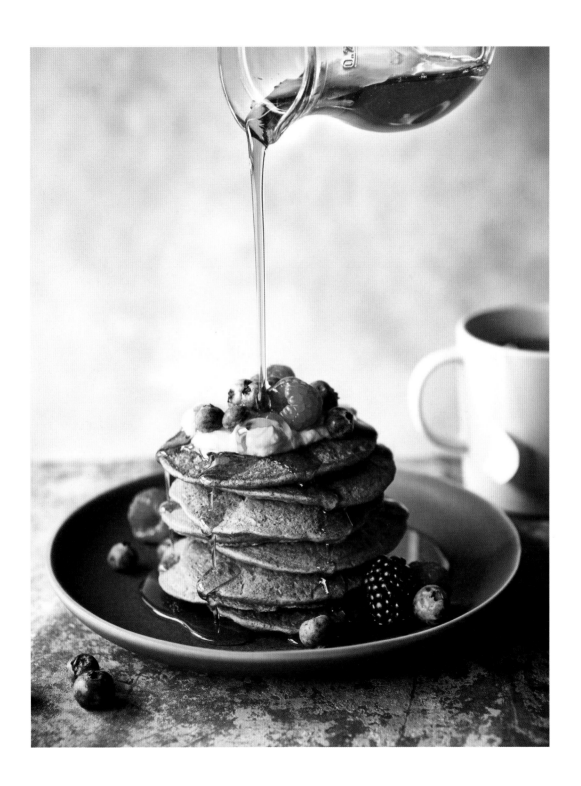

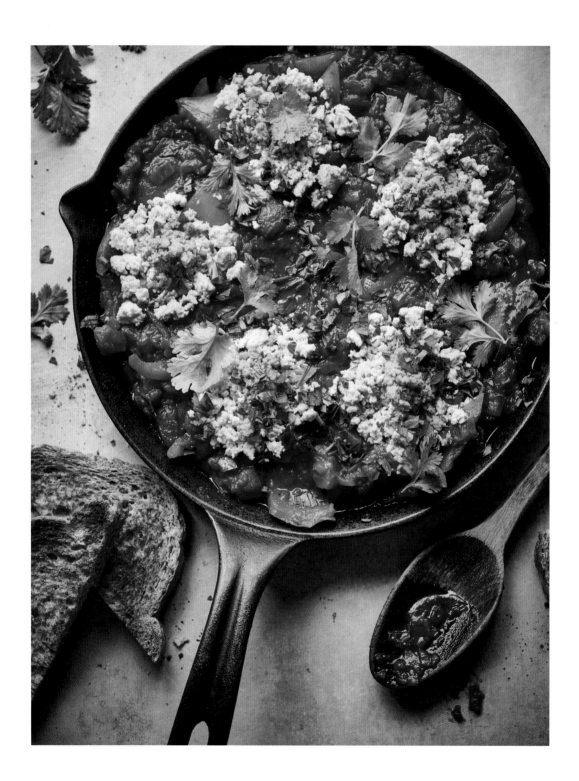

Vegan Shakshuka ♡ ⊘

Shakshuka is a Middle Eastern dish of eggs baked in a roasted pepper and tomato sauce. In our vegan version we stay true to the sauce and the baking style and add our delicious scramble in place of the traditional eggs.

Serves 4–6
Takes 40 minutes

Roasted pepper tomato sauce
2 large red onions, diced
2 red peppers, sliced
2 yellow peppers, sliced
1 teaspoon salt
½ teaspoon cumin seeds
1 teaspoon ground cumin
½ teaspoon smoked paprika
a pinch of cayenne pepper
¼ teaspoon ground black pepper
2 bay leaves
1 tablespoon tamari/soy sauce (make sure to use gf soy sauce if you need to avoid gluten)
1 tablespoon maple syrup
6 sprigs of fresh thyme
2 x 400g tins of chopped tomatoes

Easy scramble
300g firm tofu
¾ teaspoon onion powder
¼ teaspoon ground turmeric
1½ teaspoons tamari/soy sauce (make sure to use gf soy sauce if you need to avoid gluten)
⅓ teaspoon black sulphur salt or kala namak or any sea salt if you can't get this)

To serve
1 ripe avocado
30g fresh coriander, chopped
15g fresh flat-leaf parsley, chopped
sliced wholemeal bread

Preheat the oven to 180°C fan/200°C.

To make the roasted pepper tomato sauce, heat a non-stick ovenproof pan over a high heat. Once hot, add the onions, peppers and ½ teaspoon of salt, stirring regularly. Cook until the onions start to brown, then add 3 tablespoons of water, cover the pan with a lid and allow the veg to sweat for 6–8 minutes, stirring occasionally. Add the remaining ingredients for the sauce and bring to the boil. Reduce the heat to low and leave to simmer for 10 minutes, stirring occasionally.

While the veg are cooking, prepare the scramble. Drain the tofu to remove any liquid, then put in a bowl with the onion powder and mash until the tofu is crumbled. Move two thirds to a separate bowl with a pinch of salt and mix, and to the remaining third add the turmeric and tamari and mix.

Heat a non-stick pan on a medium heat. Once hot, add the bigger tofu mixture and fry, stirring continuously. If it catches, add 1 teaspoon of water to loosen. Cook for 3–4 minutes.

Take the pepper tomato sauce off the heat and remove the bay leaves. Roughly divide the white tofu mixture into 4–6 circles, then dot these around the pepper tomato sauce and spread them out slightly to create your tofu 'egg whites'.

Now, to cook the turmeric 'egg yolks': in the same pan cook the remaining tofu mix for 3–4 minutes, until it has started to turn a yellow similar to scrambled eggs. Add a dot of yellow mix on top of the tofu 'egg whites' in the sauce.

To finish, pop the dish into the preheated oven for 5 minutes.

Remove the shakshuka from the oven and garnish with the fresh coriander and flat-leaf parsley. Sprinkle the yellow tofu scramble with the black sulphur salt (this salt can lose its flavour when heated, so it's best added just before serving). Serve family style, with your toast and sliced avocado.

Breakfast

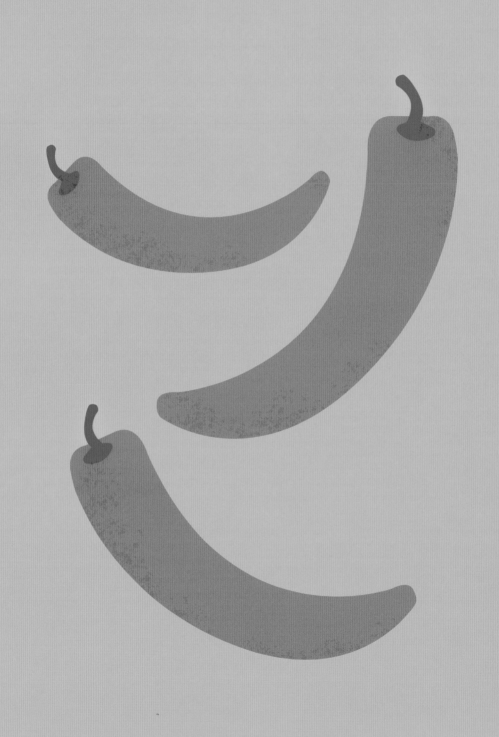

Chapter 9

Soup

A good bowl of soup can be nourishing for the soul!
We have a selection of our favourites here – some chunky,
some smooth, and all delicious!

Thai Noodle Soup ♡ ⃠

The first time we made a variation of this was with a friend called Sadia.
Here we have simplified the original recipe to give you a delicious,
warming, hearty, and frankly quite exotic soup.

Serves 4
Takes 30 minutes

Paste
1 lemongrass stalk
2 chillies, deseeded if you prefer
    less heat
2 spring onions/scallions
4 peeled cloves of garlic
a thumb-size piece of fresh ginger
1 tablespoon ground coriander
½ tablespoon ground turmeric
1 teaspoon curry powder
4 tablespoons water
1 x 400ml tin of coconut milk
    (use light if you want to be
    Happy Heart-friendly)

Soup
300g wholewheat or brown rice
    noodles
1 x 200g block of firm tofu
50g green beans
100g oyster mushrooms
1 small carrot
3 tablespoons tamari/soy sauce
    (use gf soy sauce if you avoid
    gluten)
1½ litres veg stock
2 tablespoons maple syrup

Garnish options
1 fresh red chilli
2 spring onions/scallions
1 lime
15g fresh coriander
50g roasted salted peanuts,
    chopped
20g beansprouts
¼ of a red onion

Remove and discard the fibrous first layer from the lemongrass stalk,
then roughly chop. In a blender or using a soup blender, mix the
lemongrass with the rest of the paste ingredients until smooth, adding
a little more water if needed.

Cook the noodles according to the packet instructions until slightly al
dente (ever so slightly undercooked), then drain and rinse in cold
water to stop them cooking further and to remove excess starch so
they don't stick together.

Cut the tofu into even bite-size squares, cut the green beans into
thirds, and chop the mushrooms into small bite-size pieces. Chop the
carrot into matchsticks or finely grate.

Heat a large non-stick pan on a high heat. Once hot, add the tofu,
then reduce the heat to medium and cook until nicely browned and
fried on all sides, stirring occasionally, for 3–5 minutes. If it starts to
stick to the bottom at any stage, add 1 teaspoon of water to release
it from the pan and stir. Add the tamari/soy sauce, coating all the
tofu for 1–2 minutes, and move it all around to ensure an even
coating. Remove from the pan and set aside.

Add the mushrooms and green beans to the pan along with
1 tablespoon of water. Cook, stirring occasionally, for 3 minutes,
then remove from the pan.

Add the paste to the pan and cook over a low heat, stirring
occasionally, for 4–5 minutes. Add the stock, stirring gently, bring
to the boil, then lower the heat to a simmer for 5 minutes. Add the
maple syrup and simmer for another few minutes.

While the soup is simmering, get your garnish ready. Slice the fresh
red chilli and the spring onions/scallions, quarter the lime, and
roughly chop the coriander and peanuts. Rinse the beansprouts, and
finely slice the red onion.

Put the tofu, veg and noodles back into the soup for a moment to heat
through, then divide between bowls and serve with your choice of
garnish. Perfect comfort and noodle joy in a bowl!

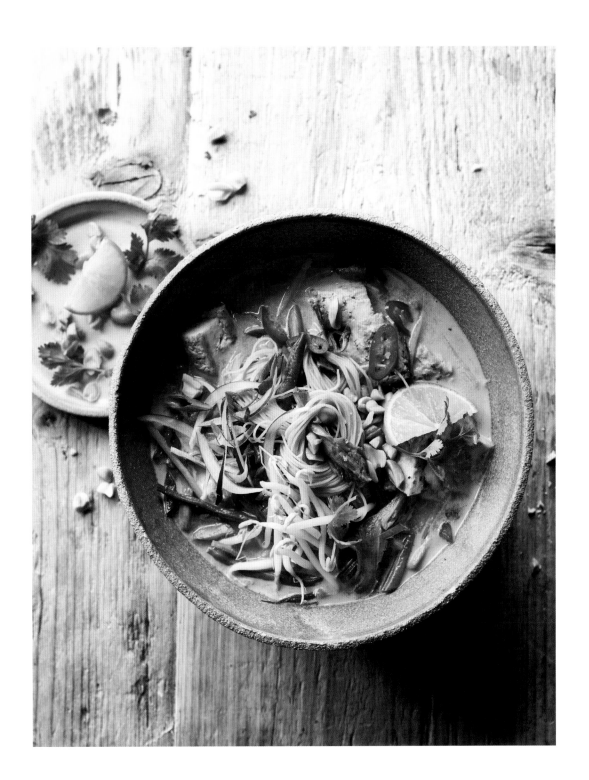

Easy Miso Soup 3 Ways ♡ ✋ ⃠

Growing up in Ireland, we often saw this Japanese dish as an exotic magical health tonic with super-nourishing properties, guaranteed to cure a hangover or at least give you a belly hug.

Serves 4
Takes 10 minutes

Miso base
1½ litres warm water
2 cloves of garlic
2½cm cube of fresh
   ginger, grated
3 tablespoons tamari/
   soy sauce (make sure to
   use gf soy sauce if you
   need to avoid gluten)
4 teaspoons/10g dried
   seaweed (kelp, kombu,
   nori, arame)
¼ teaspoon chilli powder or
   cayenne pepper
1 teaspoon dried mushroom
   powder, such as shiitake or
   porcini mushroom
   (optional)
2 tablespoons fresh miso of
   choice (white will be
   lighter and sweeter, darker
   will be stronger)

Summer veg
50g sugar snaps
50g radishes
50g cucumber

Winter veg
50g carrots
100g potatoes
a handful of spinach, to serve

Spring veg
100g firm tofu
50g shiitake mushrooms

The first thing you need to do is make your miso base. Blend 1 litre of warm water with the garlic, peeled and grated ginger and tamari/soy sauce. Roughly chop the seaweed if not using a seaweed powder.

Transfer this miso base to a medium pot and add the seaweed and the mushroom powder (or grated potato, see below), if using, along with the chilli powder/cayenne powder and the fresh miso. Bring to the boil, then reduce to a simmer for 10 minutes.

While the stock is simmering prepare your veg:

- Roughly chop the sugar snaps.

- Slice the radishes.

- Julienne the cucumber or cut into matchsticks.

- Finely grate the carrot.

- Grate the potato – this will need to be added to the miso base while it's heating, to ensure it cooks through – it will take a little longer (10 minutes) but will give you a thicker, more comforting miso, Irish style!

- Wash the spinach.

- Cut the tofu into approx. 3cm cubes.

- Cut the shiitake mushrooms into quarters.

Turn the heat off, then add your veg and stir through the miso base with a fork.

Serve in small bowls and enjoy this wonderful comforting elixir!

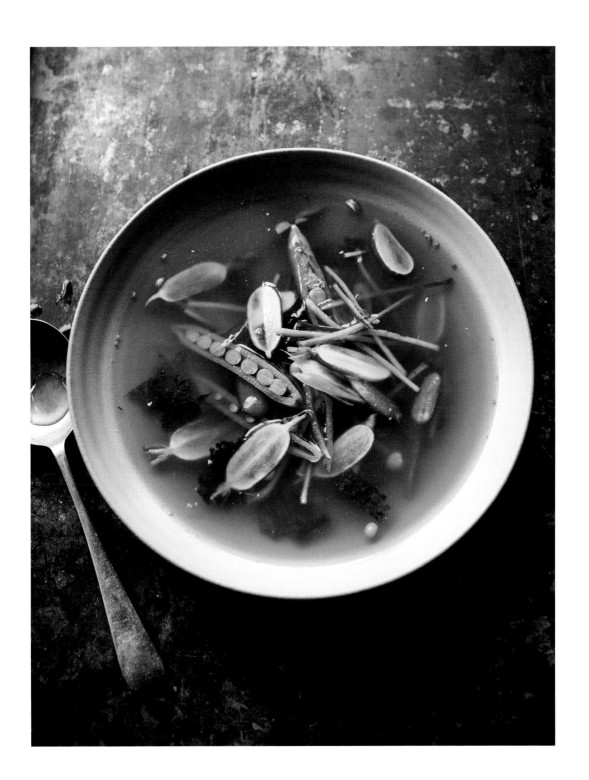

Lentil Sambar Soup ♡ ✋ ⃠ ⊜

A sambar is a warming lentil soup made with tamarind pulp, which gives it a sweet and sour note that cuts through the lentils. This soup is so delicious and nourishing – it really tastes cosy, like sitting by the fire on a cold day.

Serves 6
Takes 35 minutes

250g green tops of 2 leeks (use none of the white part, as this is high-FODMAP)
2 medium carrots (approx. 200g)
2 medium potatoes (450g)
½ a fresh red chilli
3cm piece of fresh ginger
1 teaspoon salt
1 tablespoon ground turmeric
1 tablespoon curry powder
½ teaspoon ground black pepper
1 tablespoon tamari/soy sauce (make sure to use gf soy sauce if you need to avoid gluten)
2.2 litres veg stock (see low-FODMAP recipe on page 103) or water
1 x 400g tin of chopped tomatoes
130g split red lentils
1 tablespoon tamarind pulp (or ½ tablespoon lime juice + ½ tablespoon coconut/brown sugar)
10g fresh coriander (or other fresh herb)
100g baby spinach or similar greens

Toasted seeds and spices
1 tablespoon cumin seeds
3 tablespoon sesame seeds
1 teaspoon black or yellow mustard seeds

Cut the green tops of the leeks down the centre lengthwise and give them a good wash, as sediment often hides here. Slice into thin strips. Roughly cut the carrots and potatoes into small bite-size pieces so that they will cook quickly. Finely chop the chilli (include the seeds and white membrane inside if you prefer it spicier, or leave out if you prefer it milder). Finely chop the ginger.

Put a large pot on a high heat. Once hot, add the leek greens and fry for 4 minutes, stirring continuously. If they start to stick, add ½ teaspoon of water and stir to loosen them from the bottom of the pot. Add the chopped ginger and chilli and fry for 2 minutes, stirring regularly. Add another teaspoon of water if it starts to stick again. The leeks should be starting to brown around the edges.

Add the carrots and potatoes together with the salt, turmeric, curry powder, ground black pepper and tamari/soy sauce, then add 50ml of the veg stock and stir well. Put the lid on the pot, turn the heat down to medium and leave to cook for 5 minutes, stirring occasionally.

Add the chopped tomatoes, red lentils, and the remaining veg stock or water, then add the tamarind pulp (or lime juice + sugar) and stir well. Turn the heat up to high and bring to the boil with the lid on. Once the soup boils, reduce to a simmer and leave to cook for 25 minutes, stirring regularly to ensure the lentils aren't sticking to the bottom of the pot.

While the soup is simmering, toast the spices. Heat a non-stick pan on a medium heat. Once hot, add the spices and a generous pinch of salt and fry until they start to pop, making sure you stir regularly to prevent them burning. Once they begin to pop and the sesame seeds start to go golden, turn off the heat, pour the spices into a bowl and set aside for the garnish.

Check the seasoning and add more salt, pepper or lime juice to the soup if necessary. Roughly chop the fresh coriander.

Remove the soup from the heat and add the spinach and coriander. Garnish each bowl with a generous dusting of toasted spices.

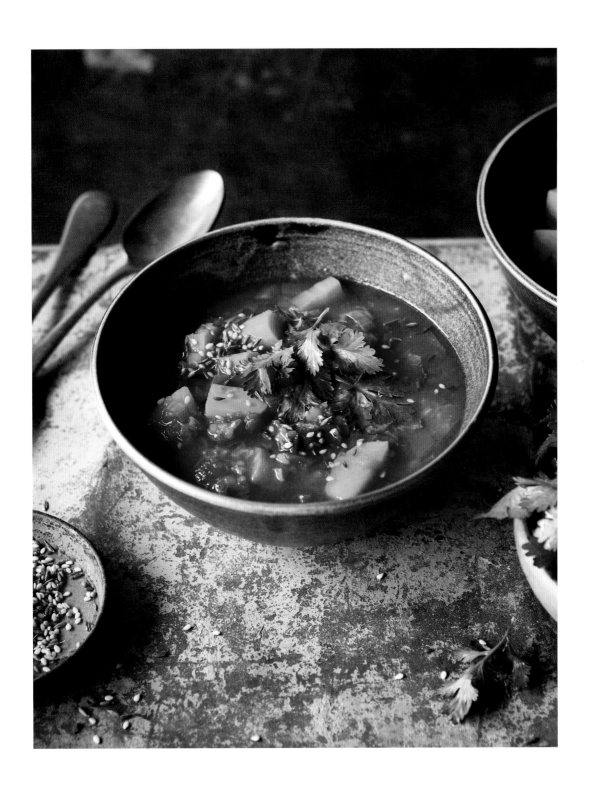

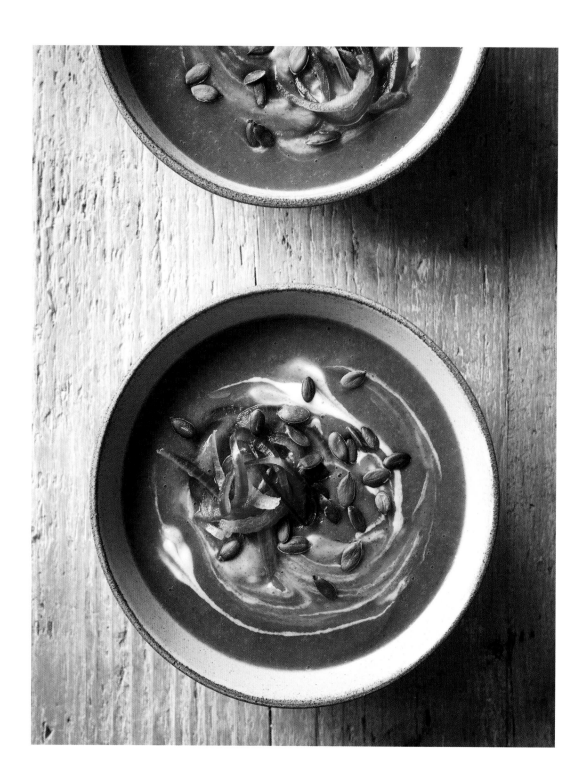

Eat Your Greens Soup ♡ ✋ ⊘ ⊜

As the name implies, this one is a great way to get more greens into you! Appropriately named by our chef mom, Dorene Palmer, many years ago, it's well worth making this a part of your weekly meals, as most of us need to eat more green veg.

Serves 6
Takes 40 minutes

400g potatoes (approx.
   2–3 medium potatoes)
300g celeriac (approx.
   ½ a celeriac)
2 leeks, green part only
   (250g) (use none of the
   white part, as this is
   high-FODMAP)
1½ teaspoons salt
2 litres veg stock (see
   low-FODMAP recipe
   on page 103)
1 bay leaf (optional)
½ teaspoon ground
   black pepper
100g baby spinach
a dash of lemon juice
   (optional)
125g coconut or soy yoghurt,
   to serve

Optional garnish
5g sauerkraut
15g pumpkin seeds

Chop the potato and celeriac into small bite-size pieces (leaving the skin on the potatoes). Give the leeks a good clean – sediment can often be hidden in the centre. We use only the green part of the leeks, as they are low-FODMAP and also more nutritious than the white part – and they give this soup a wonderful vibrant colour. (Keep the white part to use in another dish in place of an onion.) Roughly chop the leek greens.

Heat a large pot on a high heat. Once it heats up, add the prepared leeks and a pinch of salt and cook for 3 minutes, stirring regularly. If they start to stick, add 1 teaspoon of water. Next add the potato and celeriac, 50ml of veg stock and a pinch of salt, stir well, then reduce the heat to medium and put the lid on. Leave to sweat or steam for 8 minutes, stirring regularly, and again if the veg starts to stick to the bottom add a teaspoon of water and stir to loosen the veg from the pan.

Add the rest of the veg stock, with the bay leaf and black pepper. Bring to the boil, then reduce the heat to a gentle simmer and cook until the potato is nice and soft, about 15 minutes.

Remove from the heat, add the baby spinach and blend until smooth. Adjust the seasoning if needed by adding more salt and ground black pepper, or an acid such as a dash of lemon juice to taste.

Serve in bowls, with a nice swirl of coconut or soy yoghurt on top, and a garnish of pickled red onions and pumpkin seeds, if you like.

Soup

Creamed Cauliflower and Coconut Soup ♡ ✋ ⃠

Cauliflower was always one of our nemeses, growing up. We only ever ate it boiled with a cheese sauce, but once we learnt how to roast, char, fry, batter or even glaze it, we started to realize how versatile a veg it is.

Serves 5–6
Takes 40 minutes

1 head of cauliflower, including the leaves (approx. 800g)
4 medium potatoes (approx. 800g)
2 teaspoons salt
2 white onions
4 cloves of garlic
½ a thumb-size piece of fresh ginger
2 litres veg stock
1 x 400ml tin of coconut milk (full-fat, but to be Happy Heart-friendly use low-fat)
3 sprigs of fresh thyme
juice of ½ a lemon
½ teaspoon ground black pepper
a dash of vinegar (optional)

Preheat the oven to 200°C fan/220°C. Fill and boil the kettle.

Remove the leaves from the cauliflower, keeping the smaller nicer-looking ones with smaller central spines. Cut the cauliflower into rough bite-size pieces. We do this so it will cook quicker. Cut the potatoes into bite-size pieces, leaving the skin on. Put the cauliflower and potatoes into a pan, pour in 200ml of boiling water, add a generous pinch of salt, then put the lid on and bring to the boil on a high heat. Once boiling, reduce to a simmer and leave to steam for 8–10 minutes.

While the cauliflower is steaming, peel and finely dice the onions. Peel the garlic and leave whole. Peel and finely dice the ginger.

Remove the cauliflower and potatoes from the pot and drain in a colander. Divide between two baking trays along with the onions, cauliflower greens and whole garlic cloves. Add a generous pinch of salt and mix well. Make sure there is enough room for all the veg – if they are on top of each other they will steam as opposed to baking. Bake in the preheated oven for 20 minutes.

While the veg are baking, put the ginger, veg stock, coconut milk and most of the thyme leaves into a large pot and bring to the boil with the lid on. Once boiling, reduce to a simmer.

When the potatoes are soft and the cauliflower is soft and slightly charred, remove them from the oven and add them to the pot of stock, excluding the cauliflower greens. Pop these back into the oven until they have crisped up nicely – they will make a lovely garnish.

Bring the stock to the boil again and turn off the heat. Add the lemon juice and the black pepper and blend, using a hand blender, until smooth and creamy. Taste and adjust the seasoning with salt, black pepper or a dash of vinegar. Remove the cauliflower greens from the oven.

Serve the soup in bowls, with the rest of the thyme leaves and the baked cauliflower greens to garnish.

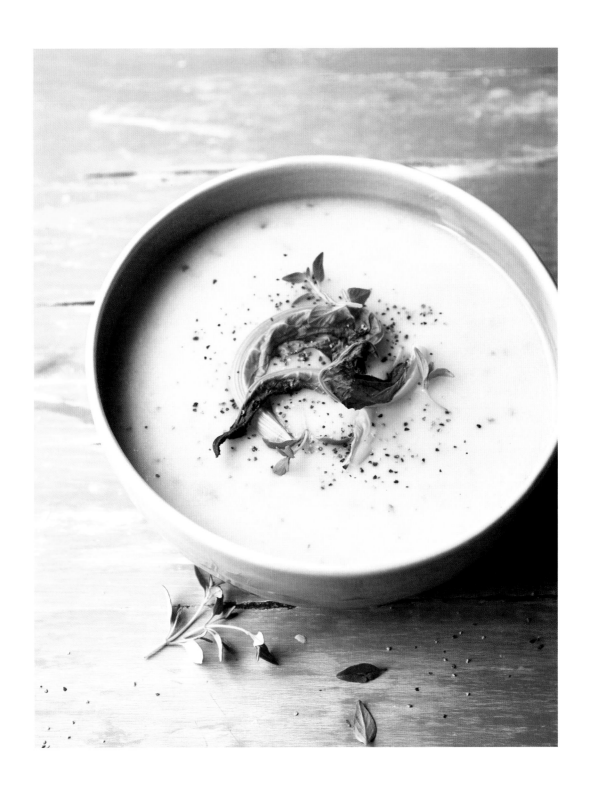

Maple Roasted Root Veg Soup ♡ ✋ ◌ ☺

Root veg are naturally sweet, one of the sweetest of all being the humble carrot. Here we roast them with a little maple syrup, to heighten the sweetness and give them a lovely glaze. When blended through the soup, they give a lovely caramel flavour and a sweet yumminess! The potato gives a great natural low-fat source of creaminess.

Serves 6
Takes 40 minutes

4 carrots (approx. 600g)
green tops of 2–3 leeks (250g) (use none of the white part, as this is high-FODMAP)
4 potatoes (800g)
1 teaspoon salt (if basing the soup on water, you will need more like 2 teaspoons, whereas if stock-based you will only need 1 teaspoon)
4 tablespoons maple syrup
6 sprigs of fresh thyme
2 litres veg stock (see low-FODMAP recipe on page 103)
2 bay leaves
½ teaspoon ground black pepper
1 tablespoon apple cider vinegar

Preheat the oven to 180°C fan/200°C.

Chop the carrots into small bite-size pieces. Slice the leeks in half lengthwise and clean them thoroughly (sand can often hide in the layers), then chop into small pieces. Cut the potatoes (leave them unpeeled) into bite-size pieces.

Put the veg into a large bowl with the salt, maple syrup and the thyme leaves, stripped from their stalks, and mix well. Add 2 tablespoons of water (this will ensure that the veg steam as well as bake).

Spread the veg evenly on two baking trays, making sure they all have enough room and are not stacked on top of each other. Bake in the preheated oven for 30 minutes, stirring once or twice to ensure they cook evenly.

Put the veg stock or water into a large pot with the bay leaves and black pepper, bring to the boil, then reduce to a simmer.

Remove the veg from the oven and check that they are all cooked through. The carrots will take the longest, so check that these are soft right through to the centre.

Remove the bay leaves from the simmering stock and add the roasted veg, along with the vinegar. Using a hand blender, blend until smooth and creamy.

Taste and adjust the seasoning with salt, black pepper, and possibly a little extra vinegar to cut through the sweetness.

Sweet Potato and Chickpea Soup ⊙ ✋ ⊘

This is a lovely smooth and sweet soup that's served with baked crispy chickpeas to give it a beautiful contrasting bite. It's great to double up this recipe when you're making it, and freeze half.

Serves 6–8
Takes 50 minutes

1 medium red onion
4 cloves of garlic
2 medium carrots
  (approx. 200g)
1 potato (approx. 200g)
a thumb-size piece of
  fresh ginger
1 teaspoon salt
1 teaspoon tamari/soy sauce
  (make sure to use gf soy
  sauce if you need to avoid
  gluten)
½ teaspoon ground
  black pepper
2½ litres veg stock/water
1kg sweet potatoes
juice of 1 lime

Baked chickpeas
1 x 400g tin of chickpeas
  (approx. 240g when
  drained)
2 tablespoons tamari/
  soy sauce (make sure to
  use gf soy sauce if you
  need to avoid gluten)
½ teaspoon smoked paprika

Preheat the oven to 200°C fan/220°C.

First, bake the chickpeas. Drain and rinse them, then place on a baking tray along with the tamari/soy sauce and smoked paprika and mix well. Bake in the preheated oven for 25 minutes, stirring once or twice.

Peel and roughly chop the onion and garlic. Roughly chop the carrots and potato, leaving the skin on the potato. Peel and finely chop the ginger.

Heat a large pan on a high heat. Once hot, add the chopped onion and ginger and fry for 4 minutes, stirring regularly. If they start to stick, add 1 teaspoon of water and stir to loosen. Cook until the onions start to brown slightly. Add the chopped garlic and fry for another minute. You may need to add another teaspoon of water to avoid everything sticking again, depending on your pot.

Next, add the carrots, potato, salt, black pepper, tamari/soy sauce and 50ml of veg stock. Give it a good stir, then put the lid on and leave for 5 minutes on a medium heat, stirring occasionally.

Chop the sweet potatoes, leaving the skin on. Add to the pan with the rest of the veg stock/water, then turn up the heat and bring to the boil. Once boiling, turn down the heat and leave to simmer for 25 minutes, until the sweet potato is soft.

Turn off the heat, squeeze in the juice of the lime and use a hand blender to blend until smooth. If the soup is too thick, add boiling water until you achieve the desired consistency.

Remove the baked chickpeas from the oven and serve some on top of each bowl of soup, for a lovely crunchy, umami smoked addition of flavour.

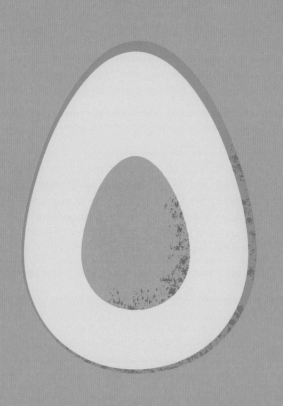

Chapter 10

Salads

Bright, bountiful and abundant. This salad section will help you redefine what a healthy salad is! We have lots of cracking salads that will work either on their own, as a meal or shared as a side.

Middle Eastern Greens Pot

Quick, tasty and full of flavour, the toasted seeds add crunch and protein, and the cumin brings in a lovely Middle Eastern musky note which is a stark contrast to the lemon and mint. Simple yet delicious. Serve with beetroot hummus, to add a vibrant colour contrast.

Serves 2–3

Takes 10 minutes (longer if cooking your own quinoa)

1 x 250g pack of cooked quinoa (or you can cook your own)
1 teaspoon ground turmeric
50g frozen peas
1 tablespoon cumin seeds
25g pumpkin seeds
10g fresh mint
zest and juice of ½ a lemon
½ teaspoon salt
100g hummus/beetroot hummus (see pages 256–7)

Fill and boil a kettle. Put the quinoa into a bowl, add the ground turmeric and mix well. In a separate bowl, pour boiling water over the frozen peas to defrost them, then drain and rinse them.

Heat a non-stick pan on a high heat. Add the cumin and pumpkin seeds and toast until they start to pop, stirring regularly – this should take somewhere between 4 and 6 minutes. Remove and set aside. Pick the mint leaves off the stalks and finely chop them.

Put the quinoa, lemon zest and juice, chopped mint and salt into a bowl and mix together. Add the frozen peas.

Serve with the hummus on the side, and garnish with lots of the toasted seeds.

Peanut Satay Tofu Pot ♡ 🤚 ⊘

These make the perfect snack, or a light lunch on the go, or can be easily fleshed out to make a delicious dinner. Here we use cooked quinoa as the base, due to its higher protein content, and add delicious salty-sweet tofu on top.

Serves 3

Takes 15 minutes (longer if cooking your own quinoa)

½ a thumb-size piece of fresh ginger
4 tablespoons peanut butter
2 tablespoons tamari/ soy sauce (make sure to use gf soy sauce if you need to avoid gluten)
2 tablespoons apple cider vinegar
2 tablespoons maple syrup
250g firm tofu
1 x 250g pack of cooked quinoa (or you can cook your own)
1 medium carrot
2 spring onions/scallions
1 teaspoon salt
¼ teaspoon ground black pepper
juice of ½ a lime
4 tablespoons toasted peanuts
10g fresh coriander or parsley

Peel and finely grate the ginger. Mix together the peanut butter, 200 ml warm water, tamari/soy sauce, vinegar, ginger and maple syrup until it's nice and smooth. Cut the tofu into squares approx. 4cm x 4cm and 2cm thick.

Heat a non-stick pan on a high heat. Once hot, add the tofu squares and cook for 3–4 minutes on each side until they start to turn brown or golden. Add half the peanut sauce and move it around the pan quickly to ensure all the tofu is well coated on both sides. Leave to cook for a further minute on each side, then remove the tofu from the pan and set aside.

Put the quinoa into a large bowl. Grate the carrot, finely slice the spring onions/scallions, and add these to the cooked quinoa along with the salt, black pepper and lime juice. Mix well. Divide the quinoa between three bowls, pour the remaining sauce on top and mix slightly. Serve with 2 slices of tofu per person, sprinkled with toasted peanuts and fresh coriander. Serve a little of the remaining sauce on the side.

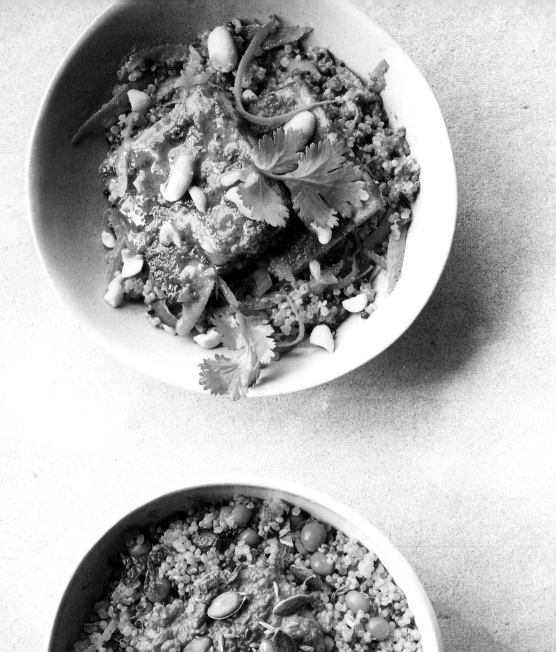
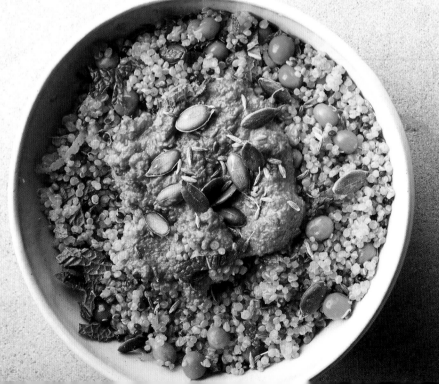

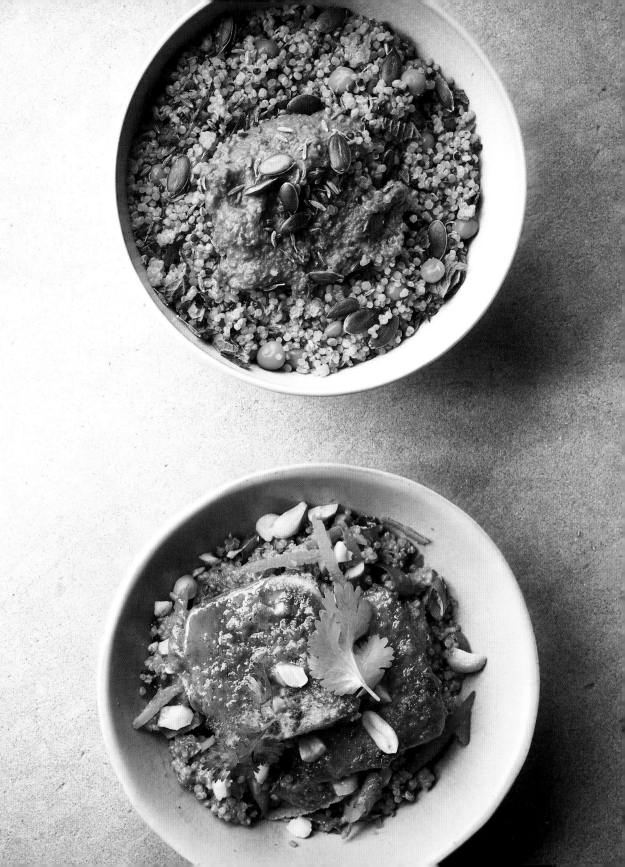

Japanese Teriyaki Tofu and Grain Bowl ♡ ⊛ ⊘

Inspired by light and yet umami-packed Japanese cooking, this salad has a great variety of texture and colour. If you want to be gluten-free, just replace the couscous with quinoa or brown rice.

Serves 4
Takes 15 minutes

200g wholemeal couscous/400g cooked brown rice or quinoa
2 tablespoons tamari/soy sauce (make sure to use gf soy sauce if you need to avoid gluten)
150g frozen peas
400g firm tofu
40g sesame seeds
1 avocado
1 fresh red chilli
100g sauerkraut (ideally red, if you can find it)

Teriyaki sauce

1 tablespoon maple syrup
1 teaspoon mirin (optional)
½ a thumb-size piece of fresh ginger
4 tablespoons tamari/soy sauce (make sure to use gf soy sauce if you need to avoid gluten)

Fill and boil a kettle. If using couscous, put it into a medium bowl with the tamari/soy sauce and mix well. Level out the couscous, then pour over enough boiling water to cover it by 1cm. Cover with a plate and leave to soak for 5 minutes. Once it's ready, use a fork to fluff it up. If using brown rice or quinoa, just put it into the bowl with the tamari/soy sauce.

Put the frozen peas into a second bowl and cover with boiling water. Leave to thaw. Peel and finely dice the fresh ginger and in a mug, mix together the ingredients for the teriyaki sauce.

Take the tofu from the pack and press it firmly to remove any excess moisture. Slice it into squares about 4cm x 4cm and 2cm thick. Heat a non-stick wide-based pan on a high heat. Once hot, add the sliced tofu so that it makes a single layer in the pan and cook until it starts to brown on both sides – this should take about 3–4 minutes each side. Once brown on both sides, add the teriyaki sauce to the pan. It will sizzle and make a noise, but don't worry. Spread the sauce around quickly, as it will want to stick. After 30 seconds/1 minute, once the sauce has evaporated, flip the tofu and cook for another 30 seconds/1 minute. Remove the tofu from the pan.

Add 2 tablespoons of water to deglaze the pan, stirring in any charred or sticky bits, and set the liquid aside. Clean and dry the pan, then put it back on a high heat. Once hot, add the sesame seeds and toast for 4–5 minutes until they start to pop, stirring regularly to prevent them burning.

Add the deglazed sauce to the couscous or rice to give it more base flavour, and mix well.

Drain and rinse the peas. Cut the avocado into quarters, removing the stone, and use a spoon to remove the flesh from the skin. Finely slice the red chilli, leaving the seeds in if you like it hot.

Divide the couscous between four bowls, followed by the sauerkraut, peas, avocado, and finally the teriyaki tofu. Garnish with the sesame seeds and the red chilli slices.

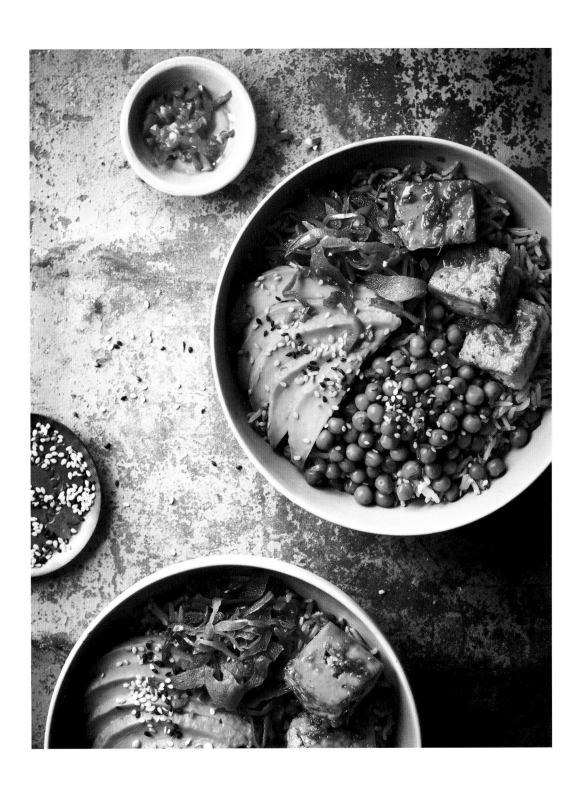

Lebanese Lemon Parsley Bean Salad ♡ ✋ ⊘

This salad is easy to make, fresh, wholefood, and when served with toasted pitta bread it becomes like the famous Lebanese fattoush salad. It is great served with a generous serving of hummus (see page 256).

Serves 4–6
Takes 15 minutes

3 cloves of garlic
25g fresh flat-leaf or
    curly parsley
25g fresh mint
1 small red onion (120g)
1 cucumber (approx. 300g)
10 ripe cherry tomatoes
1 yellow pepper
    (approx. 200g)
1 x 400g tin of butter beans
    (approx. 240g when
    drained)
1 x 400g tin of kidney beans
    (approx. 240g when
    drained)
1 x 400g tin of chickpeas
    (approx. 240g when
    drained)
juice of 2 lemons
2 teaspoons salt
1 teaspoon paprika
1 tablespoon sumac
¼ teaspoon chilli powder/
    cayenne pepper
½ tablespoon ground cumin

Serving suggestions
4 wholemeal pitta breads or
    gluten-free pitta breads
a big dollop of hummus (see
    page 256)
sriracha sauce (see
    page 187)

Peel and finely chop the garlic. Remove the parsley and mint leaves from their stalks and finely chop them.

Peel the red onion and slice it into thin long strips. Cut the cucumber into 1½cm cubes. Chop the cherry tomatoes into quarters and cut the yellow pepper into thin squares about 2cm x 2cm.

Drain and rinse the three tins of beans, then put all the ingredients into a large bowl and mix well.

If serving with pitta bread, toast the pittas and rip them up to serve with the salad, along with a generous dollop of hummus – and if you like it spicy, some sriracha sauce goes magic!

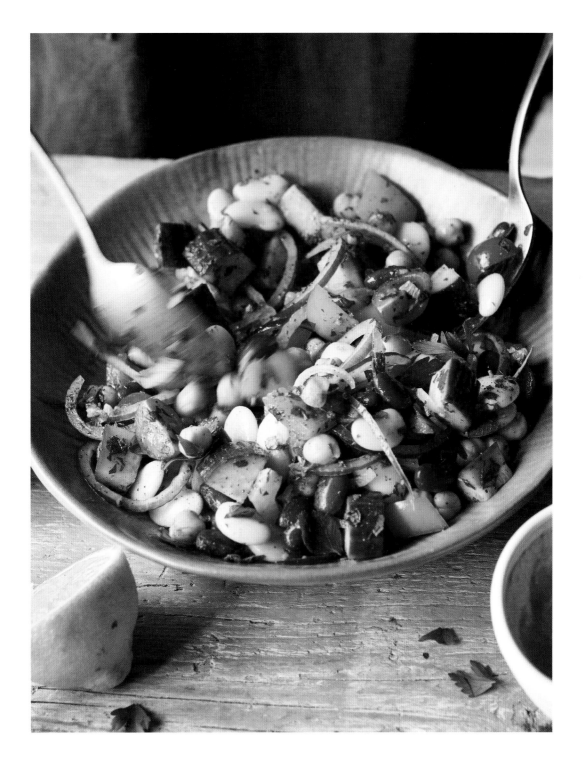

Umami Greens and Noodle Salad ♡ ✋ ◌

The closest translation of the Japanese word umami is 'delicious'. It's found in some raw tomatoes and mushrooms, but is more easily experienced in the form of soy sauce, tamari or miso.

Serves 3–4
Takes 20 minutes

200g broccoli
1½ litres veg stock
200g wholewheat or brown rice noodles
2 cloves of garlic
½ a thumb-size piece of fresh ginger
1 medium leek (250g)
1 medium courgette (200g)
100g baby spinach
25g sesame seeds (black or white)

Miso glazed tofu
200g firm tofu
1½ tablespoons miso
1½ tablespoons maple syrup

Dressing
4 tablespoons tamari/ soy sauce (make sure to use gf soy sauce if you need to avoid gluten)
1½ tablespoon maple syrup
juice of 1 lime
100ml veg stock
a pinch of salt

Cut the broccoli into bite-size florets, using as much of the stalk as you can. Bring the stock to the boil in a large saucepan, then reduce to a simmer. Add the noodles and broccoli and cook according to the noodle packet instructions. Once cooked, drain (keeping about 50ml of this veg stock), then rinse with cold water until cool, to stop further cooking. Set aside to drain again.

Peel and finely chop the garlic and ginger. Cut the leek in half lengthwise and rinse it thoroughly. Cut into pieces about 5cm long, being careful that they don't fall apart. Cut the courgette into bite-size pieces.

Heat a large non-stick pan on a high heat. Once hot, add the courgette and fry until it starts to brown – it should take about 4 minutes per side. If it starts to stick, add a teaspoon of water and stir to loosen from the pan. Add the ginger and garlic and cook for a further 2 minutes. Add the leek and the 50ml of reserved veg stock, then put a lid on the pan and leave to steam for 5 minutes. Turn off the heat, add the spinach and continue to cook with the lid on.

While the leek and spinach are cooking, heat a non-stick pan on a high heat. Once hot, add the sesame seeds and leave for a few minutes until they start to pop. Remove them from the pan and set aside.

Cut the tofu into squares approx. 4cm x 4cm and 2cm thick. Mix together the miso, maple syrup and water in a cup. Heat up the pan you used to toast the sesame seeds and add the tofu, searing it for 4–5 minutes on each side until it starts to brown. Once brown, add the miso mixture and quickly move the tofu around, flipping it so it starts to glaze and gets nice and golden on both sides. Take it off the heat, remove the tofu and set aside. Add 2 tablespoons of water to the pan and stir to remove any sauce that's sticking – put this into a small bowl with all the dressing ingredients and mix well.

Put the noodles and broccoli into a bowl along with the steamed greens, then add the dressing and mix well. Decorate with the toasted sesame seeds and serve with the tofu on top.

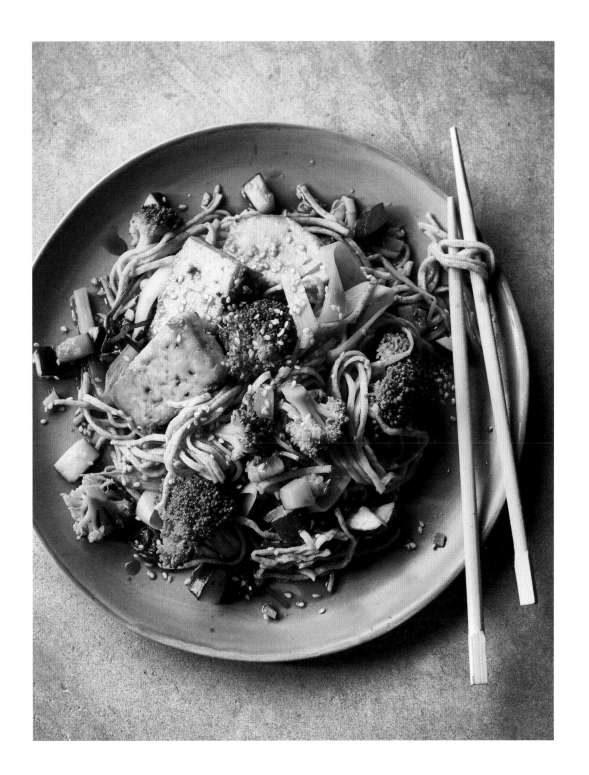

10-minute Creamy Bean and Grain Salad ♡ 🤚 ◌ 🖐

A whopping salad that can look a little ordinary, but once you start eating, the hidden sun-dried tomatoes and pickled red onions and herbs really help make it pop and sparkle.

Serves 5
Takes 10–15 minutes

50g sun-dried tomatoes (not in oil)
2 tablespoons dried mixed herbs
1 teaspoon salt
ground black pepper
150g dried wholemeal
    couscous/300g cooked
    quinoa
50g pumpkin seeds
1 medium carrot
1 bulb of fennel (approx. 260g)
100g cherry tomatoes
25g fresh basil
25g fresh flat-leaf parsley
    or coriander
1 x 400g tin of kidney beans
    (approx. 240g when drained)
1 x 400g tin of cannellini beans
    (approx. 240g when drained)

Pickled red onions
1 red onion (120g)
50ml apple cider vinegar
50ml cold water

Creamy mustard dressing
100g drained tinned
    cannellini beans
50ml lemon juice
150g coconut yoghurt/natural
    soy yoghurt
a pinch of salt and ground
    black pepper
2 teaspoons Dijon mustard

First step, let's make the pickled red onions. Peel the red onion and cut it into thin slices. Mix together the apple cider vinegar and cold water and pour over the red onion slices to pickle them. Leave them to sit for 5 minutes. Meanwhile, fill and boil a kettle.

Using scissors, chop the sun-dried tomatoes into small bite-size pieces. Put them into a bowl and stir in the mixed herbs, salt and black pepper. If using couscous, add it to the bowl and pour in enough boiling water to cover the couscous by 3cm. Cover with a plate and leave to soak for 5 minutes. Once it's ready, use a fork to fluff it up. If using cooked quinoa, just add it to the bowl of sun-dried tomatoes and leave out the soaking step.

Heat a non-stick frying pan on a high heat and add the pumpkin seeds. Leave for 5–7 minutes, until they start to pop, then take off the heat and remove the seeds from the pan.

Grate the carrot and fennel. Quarter the cherry tomatoes. Remove the basil leaves from the stalks and set aside. Roughly chop the flat-leaf parsley or coriander. Drain and rinse the beans.

To make the dressing, put all the ingredients into a blender and blend until smooth and creamy.

Drain the pickled red onions (keep the brine in the fridge for future pickling).

To serve, put the couscous/quinoa, grated carrot and fennel, beans, fresh herbs and dressing into a large bowl. Mix well, and top with the pickled onions and pumpkin seeds.

Asian Broccoli Salad in a Sweet Smoky Chilli Sauce ♡ ✋ ◇

This is a simple and super-tasty salad with great texture. The addition of the smoky toasted nuts gives a lot more depth and flavour to this dish. As the dressing is water-based, just stir it through if it starts to collect at the bottom of the dish.

Serves 4 as a lunch salad
Takes 20 minutes

300g broccoli
300g green beans
1 red pepper
100g pack of baby corn
30g pecan nuts/
   macadamia nuts
130g pack of beansprouts
20g sesame seeds

Dressing
50ml tamari/soy sauce (make
   sure to use gf soy sauce if
   you need to avoid gluten)
1½ tablespoon maple syrup
juice of 1 lime
100ml veg stock
a pinch of salt
1 tablespoon paprika
a pinch of cayenne pepper/
   chilli powder
3 tablespoons maple syrup
2 tablespoon water
juice of 1 lemon

Chop the broccoli into bite-size florets. Top and tail the green beans. Slice the red pepper into long thin strips, removing the seeds. Roughly chop the baby corn and the pecan/macadamia nuts. Rinse the beansprouts.

Steam the broccoli and the green beans over a pan of boiling water for 3 minutes, or until soft to bite, then drain in a colander and run the beans under cold running water until cool. Cut the beans in half.

Toast the sesame seeds and pecan/macadamia nuts in a frying pan on a medium heat until lightly coloured (about 5 minutes).

Put the broccoli and the rest of the salad ingredients, apart from the sesame seeds and nuts, into a large bowl. Mix together all the ingredients for the dressing, and pour over the salad. Add the sesame seeds and nuts just before serving.

Top tip: just dress what you are going to eat, as once dressed this salad will only keep for a few hours.

Vegan Caesar Salad ♡ ⓦ ◌

Here we make a few adjustments to the classic recipe to make it plant-based. If you can source tempeh it's really worth including it to make some 'facon' (fake bacon – which is delicious). For a lighter salad use soy yoghurt in the dressing, and for a more indulgent, authentic salad use store-bought vegan mayo.

Serves 4

Takes 30 minutes

150g tempeh
1 x 400g tin of chickpeas (approx. 240g when drained)
1 tablespoon gram flour or gluten-free flour
1 tablespoon tamari/ soy sauce (make sure to use gf soy sauce if you need to avoid gluten)
½ teaspoon smoked paprika
3 baby gem lettuces (600g)
100g kale
50g capers, removed from their brine (keep the brine)

Tempeh marinade
4 tablespoons tamari/soy sauce (make sure to use gf soy sauce if you need to avoid gluten)
2 tablespoons apple cider vinegar
2 tablespoons water
2 teaspoons maple syrup
2 teaspoons smoked paprika
3 tablespoons tomato purée
1 teaspoon garlic powder
a pinch of salt

Dressing
100ml soy yoghurt (use vegan mayo if following the Happy Skin plan)
15ml caper brine (see above)
a pinch of ground black pepper

Preheat the oven to 200°C fan/220°C.

Slice the tempeh into thin strips, approx. 3mm thick. Mix the ingredients for the tempeh marinade in a bowl, then add the sliced tempeh and mix well. Place on a baking tray, ensuring each piece of tempeh is well covered with the marinade, then bake for 10 minutes. Remove, turn the tempeh, and bake again for 15 minutes.

Drain and rinse the chickpeas and put them into a bowl. Sieve in the gram flour or gluten-free flour, add the tamari/soy sauce and smoked paprika, and mix well. Transfer to a baking tray and bake in the preheated oven for 20 minutes while the tempeh is cooking. Remove both the tempeh and chickpeas from the oven and leave to cool. Once the tempeh has cooled, use scissors to slice it into thin pieces about 2cm x 2cm.

Cut the base off the baby gem lettuces and peel off the leaves. Rip them up into smaller pieces and put them into a large bowl. If you want the lettuce to last longer, cut it using a plastic knife (as this reduces oxidation or browning). Rip the kale leaves from their stalks, then roughly rip them up and add to the bowl. Remove the capers from their brine, making sure to keep the brine for the dressing.

Mix together the ingredients for the dressing. Put the baby gem and kale leaves, the drained capers and dressing into a large bowl and mix well. Sprinkle over the tempeh and chickpeas and serve. Make sure the 'facon' and baked chickpeas are not mixed with the salad dressing and that they sit on the top of the salad like little flavour bombs, waiting to be enjoyed!

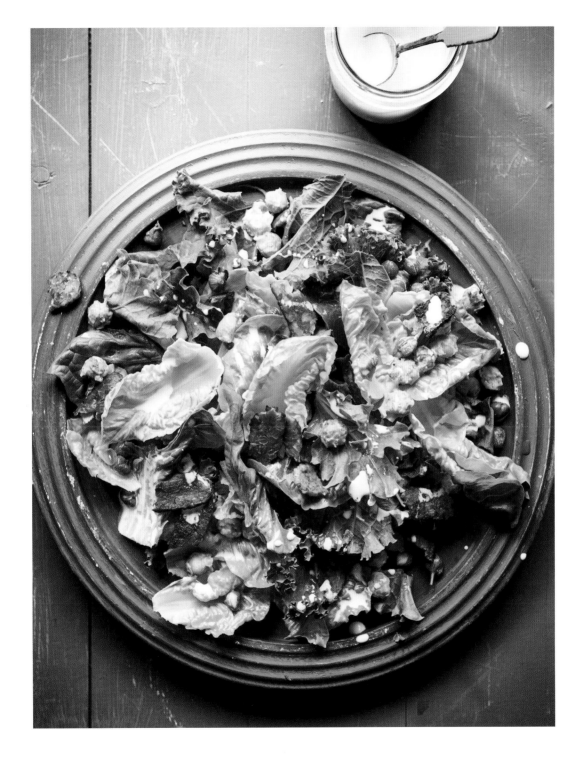

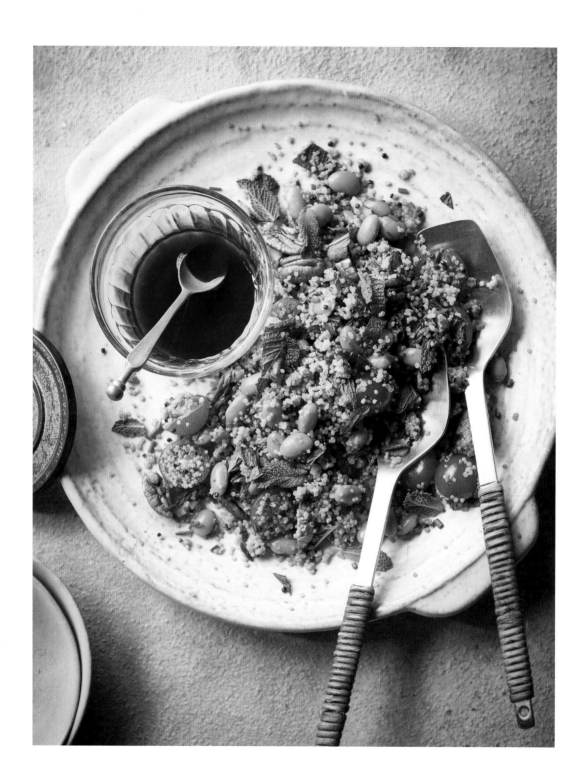

Happy Gut High Protein Quinoa Salad ♡ 🖐 ◌ 🍽

This delicious salad is super-easy to make, high in protein and is a great post-exercise meal. Packed with colour and texture, it's a bowl full of goodness that will keep your tummy happy too!

Serves 4
Takes 30 minutes

Salad
300g quinoa
60g frozen edamame beans/
   frozen peas
15 cherry tomatoes
a handful of mixed salad
   leaves
100g pecan nuts/walnuts
15g fresh mint leaves
10g fresh chives

Dressing
2½ tablespoons tamari/
   soy sauce (make sure to
   use gf soy sauce if you
   need to avoid gluten)
1 teaspoon maple syrup
2 tablespoons lemon juice
½ teaspoon salt
½ teaspoon ground
   black pepper

Cook the quinoa in 600ml of water in a pot on a high heat. Bring to the boil with the lid on, and once it boils, move the lid a little so that the steam can escape and simmer until all the water has evaporated. Remove from the heat and leave to one side with the lid on for 5–10 minutes, until the quinoa puffs up. Allow the quinoa to cool fully before mixing the salad.

Defrost the edamame beans/peas by leaving them to sit in a bowl of warm water for 10 minutes, then drain and rinse them. Cut the cherry tomatoes in half. Whisk the dressing ingredients together in a cup using a fork, or in a jug using a whisk.

Put all the salad ingredients into a large bowl and pour over the dressing.

Top tip: if you are making this ahead of time, we recommend adding the dressing just before you serve it, as it will keep better this way.

Dressings and Salad Sauces

Salad sauces might sound like a funny new phrase, but in essence the difference between salad dressings and sauces is that sauces are cooked and dressings are uncooked. Dressings are normally based on oil and vinegar and are called vinaigrettes. We wanted to move away from the traditional oil-based dressings, so we've entered more into the area of salad sauces and oil-free dressings. Use them to dress prepared raw veg, or cooked beans or legumes, to make a dressed salad, seasoning to taste.

Hoisin Sauce ♡ 🖐 ⃠

This thick, strong, full-bodied sauce originates from China, and is often used as a glazing sauce or for adding to stir-fries, or as a dipping sauce. We love to use it for noodle salads, stir-fry style salads or as a dipping sauce for raw veg or roasted veggies.

Makes approx. 125ml
Takes 5 minutes

3 tablespoons tahini (light tahini is lighter in flavour)
5 tablespoons water
1 tablespoon miso paste
3 teaspoons coconut sugar
1 teaspoon Chinese 5-spice
½ teaspoon chilli powder
2 tablespoons rice wine vinegar
2 tablespoons tamari/ soy sauce (make sure to use gf soy sauce if you need to avoid gluten)

Either whisk together the ingredients in a bowl or blend in a blender until smooth.

This makes a strong-tasting salad dressing for anything you want to give a Chinese twist to, but also goes great as a marinade for tofu, tempeh, jackfruit or mushrooms.

Sriracha Sauce ♡ 🖐 🚫

Hot, sweet and makes everything taste lovely provided you like it spicy!
This 5-minute version beats the original store-bought version in blind
taste tests. Takes sandwiches, burgers or salads to the next spicy level!

Makes approx. 350ml
Takes 5 minutes

240g fresh red chillies
50g caster sugar or
    coconut sugar
½ teaspoon salt
3 cloves of garlic
65ml apple cider vinegar
1 tablespoon sparkling water
1½ tablespoons arrowroot
    powder (or cornflour/
    tapioca flour/normal flour)

When preparing the chillies, include the green tops but remove the
stalks. Put the chillies, sugar, salt and peeled garlic into a blender and
blend until smooth. Add the vinegar, sparkling water and arrowroot
powder and blend until it is lovely and smooth.

Strain through a mesh strainer over a medium pan, pressing the pulp to
extract all the liquid.

Bring to the boil, then reduce to a gentle simmer for 5–6 minutes, stirring
regularly to avoid burning and to allow the sauce to thicken. Allow to
cool, then store in a sterilized jar.

Creamy Roasted Red Pepper Sauce ♡ 🖐 🚫

This makes a wonderful salad dressing for a leafy or grain-based
salad, and goes great with pasta, cooked veg – and most foods,
for that matter!

Makes approx. 250ml
*Takes 10 minutes (plus
soaking time)*

30g cashew nuts, soaked
    overnight (or soaked
    in boiling water for
    10 minutes)
100ml oat milk
⅓ teaspoon salt
a pinch of ground
    black pepper
a pinch of garlic powder
1 teaspoon lemon juice
1 teaspoon maple syrup
30g roasted red peppers
    (from a jar), drained

Put all the ingredients into a blender and blend until super-smooth.

This sauce will keep for 3 days in the fridge.

Salads

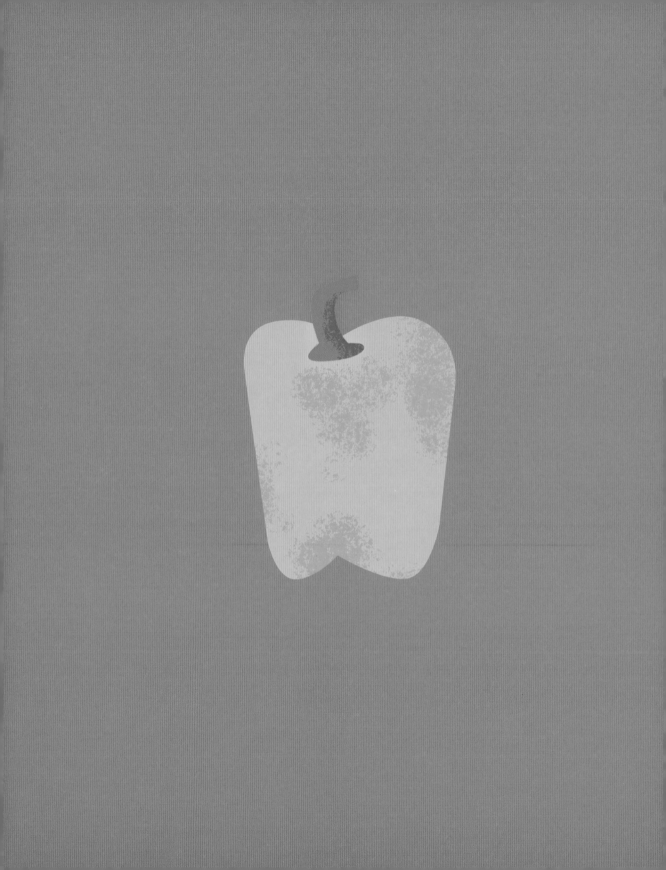

Chapter 11

Fancier Lunches

Some really lovely options here – Mexican burrito bowl, vegan hoisin 'duck' pancakes and grilled veggie and tofu kebabs, to name just a few. Whether you are enjoying a slightly fancier lunch with friends or simply treating yourself, we've got you covered here!

Burrito Bowl ♡ ✋ ⊘

This is a wonderful combination of flavours, colours and textures. It makes a great sharing plate or spread, and a delicious lunch or dinner.

Serves 4–5
Takes 30 minutes

Chocolate bean chilli
1 small red onion
3 cloves of garlic
1 fresh green chilli
100g mushrooms
1 red pepper
1 yellow pepper
1 x 400g tin of black beans (approx. 240g when drained)
1 tablespoon ground cumin
1 teaspoon cumin seeds
1 tablespoon ground coriander
½ teaspoon smoked paprika
1 teaspoon salt
a pinch of ground black pepper
2 teaspoons cocoa powder
1 x 400g tin of chopped tomatoes
1 teaspoon maple syrup
juice of 1 lime

Burrito chips
3 wholemeal burrito wraps

Guacamole
1 ripe avocado
¼ of a red onion
1 clove of garlic
4 cherry tomatoes
a pinch of salt and ground black pepper
juice of ½ a lime

Salsa
¼ of a cucumber
10 cherry tomatoes
15g fresh coriander
60g tinned sweetcorn
¼ teaspoon salt
a pinch of ground black pepper

Couscous
200g wholemeal couscous
1 teaspoon smoked paprika
1 tablespoon tamari/soy sauce (make sure to use gf soy sauce if you need to avoid gluten)

Preheat the oven to 200°C fan/220°C.

First, let's make the chocolate chilli. Peel and finely dice the red onion, garlic and chilli (leave the seeds in if you like it a little spicier). Roughly chop the mushrooms. Slice the peppers into small bite-size pieces. Drain and rinse the beans.

Heat a large non-stick pan on a high heat and add the onions, mushrooms and peppers. Fry for 8 minutes, stirring regularly, until the onions start to brown and the peppers start to soften. Add the garlic and chilli and cook for 2 minutes. Add the beans, spices, salt, black pepper and cocoa, mix well, and cook for 2 minutes. Add the chopped tomatoes, maple syrup and lime juice and bring to the boil, then reduce the heat and leave to simmer for 5 minutes.

For the burrito chips, stack the 4 wraps on top of each other and slice each of them into 8 equal triangles. Spread out on two baking trays, and bake in the preheated oven for 5 minutes on each side. Remove from the oven and leave to cool.

For the guacamole, cut the avocado in half and scoop out the flesh. Cut into small cubes and put them into a small bowl. Peel and finely dice the red onion and garlic, quarter the cherry tomatoes, and add these to the avocado. Add the salt, black pepper and lime juice, then mix well and mash. If you like a chunky guacamole, just bring everything together, but if you prefer a smooth guacamole, mash very finely.

For the salsa, chop the cucumber into 2cm cubes and quarter the cherry tomatoes. Finely chop the coriander. Mix together in a bowl along with the sweetcorn, salt and pepper.

Put the couscous into a large bowl with the smoked paprika and tamari/soy sauce, and mix well. Level out the couscous, then pour over enough boiling water to cover it by about 1cm. Cover with a plate and leave for soak for 5 minutes. Once it's ready, use a fork to fluff it up.

Divide everything between four bowls and serve.

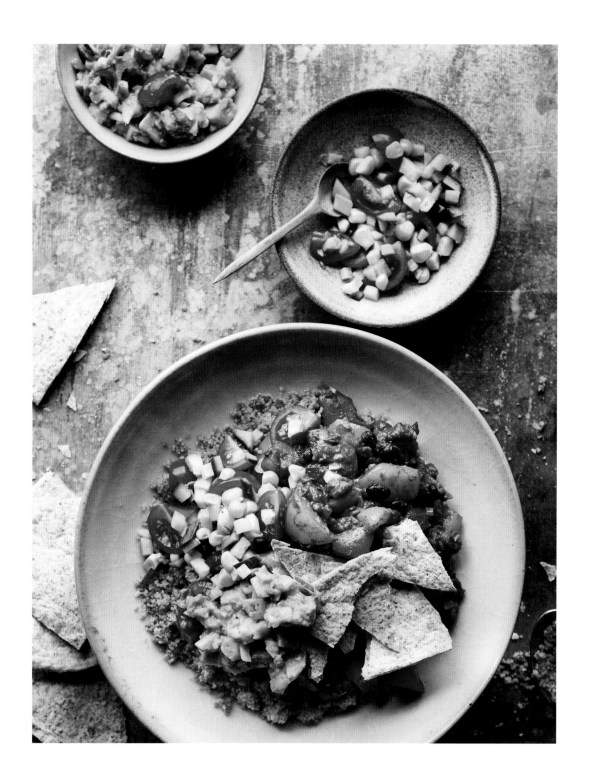

Vegan Hoisin 'Duck' Pancakes ♡ 🖐 ⊘

Here we re-create Steve's old favourite, using underripe jackfruit as the carrier for the wonderful hoisin flavour. It crisps up lovely when baked in the oven and contrasts so well with the soft, gentle Chinese-style pancakes. These are pretty simple to make, and it's a recipe you will hopefully turn to on many a day, as they are so tasty.

Serves 2
(3 pancakes each)
Takes 30 minutes

1 x 400g tin of jackfruit

Hoisin marinade
3 tablespoons tahini
5 tablespoons water
1 tablespoon miso paste
3 teaspoons brown sugar
1 teaspoon Chinese 5-spice
½ teaspoon chilli powder
2 tablespoons rice
  wine vinegar
2 tablespoons tamari/
  soy sauce (make sure to
  use gf soy sauce if you
  need to avoid gluten)

Pancakes
150g plain white flour
300ml water
2 teaspoons ground flax
  seeds

Garnish
½ a medium cucumber
3 spring onions/scallions
1 small fresh red chilli
sesame seeds

Preheat the oven to 180°C fan/200°C.

Drain the jackfruit and chop into small pieces. Put it into a bowl. Whisk all the hoisin marinade ingredients together in a medium bowl, then add three-quarters of the mixture to the jackfruit and mix well, making sure all the jackfruit is coated with the marinade. Set aside to marinate while you make the pancake batter.

Put all the pancake ingredients into a blender and blend for 30 seconds until smooth. Set aside for 2–3 minutes to allow the flax seeds to thicken.

Put the marinated jackfruit on a baking tray and spread it out into a single even layer – this will allow the edges to get crispy. Bake in the preheated oven for 20 minutes.

While the jackfruit is baking, prepare the cucumber and spring onions/scallions. Cut the cucumber into long thin 10cm strips and slice the spring onions/scallions finely at an angle. Do the same with the chilli, removing the seeds if you prefer it less hot.

To make the pancakes, heat a medium non-stick pan on a high heat. When it's hot, add a thin layer of batter, enough to make a 15cm pancake (roughly 40–50ml). Reduce the heat to medium, allow the pancake to cook for about 1 minute, then, using a silicone spatula, carefully turn it over and cook for a further minute. Continue to cook all the pancakes in batches until all the batter is used. Keep the cooked pancakes hot, wrapped in foil, while you do this.

Now it is time to build our delicious hoisin pancakes. Lay your pancakes on a plate or board and add a teaspoon of the remaining hoisin sauce to each one, along with 2–3 tablespoons of jackfruit. Add 3 or 4 strips of cucumber to each pancake, sprinkle with spring onions/scallions, chillies and sesame seeds, then wrap and enjoy!

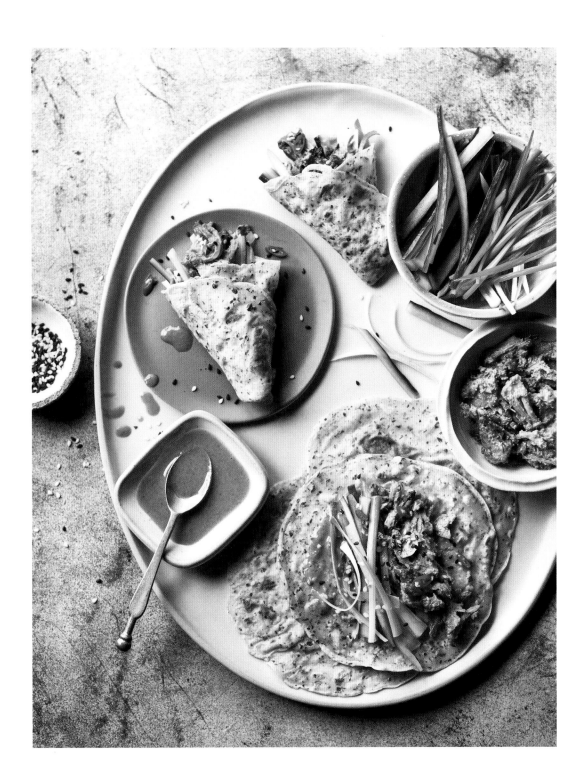

Fritters 3 Ways

Crispy, soft and gooey in the centre, these make wonderful snacks, starters and lunches, and can form a great centrepiece served with lots of salads. A fritter is generally a coated fried vegetable – here we make them lighter and healthier by using less oil and baking them.

Sweet Potato Fritters ♡ ✋ ⊘

Super-tasty, sweet and savoury, these make a fab picnic dish. These little beauties are crisp on the outside and soft and sweet on the inside. They're quick to make and they keep for 3 days in the fridge... but you will defo eat them before that!

Makes 18 small (50g) fritters
Takes approx. 50 minutes

Fritters
1kg sweet potatoes
1 fresh red chilli
2 cloves of garlic
1 red onion
1 x 400g tin of chickpeas (approx. 240g when drained)
½ teaspoon smoked paprika
½ teaspoon cumin seeds
1 teaspoon ground cumin
½ teaspoon ground black pepper
1 teaspoon salt
3 tablespoons tamari/soy sauce (make sure to use gf soy sauce if you need to avoid gluten)
juice of ½ a lemon
100g frozen peas

Batter
100g gram flour
200ml water
a pinch of salt
a pinch of ground black pepper

Preheat the oven to 180°C fan/200°C.

Chop the sweet potato into small cubes and place on a baking tray. Bake in the preheated oven for 30 minutes, then remove them, keeping the oven on.

Finely chop the chilli, garlic and red onion.

Once the sweet potatoes are baked, put them into a large bowl with the rest of the fritter ingredients apart from the peas. Using a potato masher, mash until well mixed. Add the peas and mix gently, trying to keep them whole for colour and texture.

Roll the mixture into small balls (approx. 50g each) and put them on a plate.

Sieve the gram flour into a small bowl. Add the water, salt and pepper and mix until smooth.

Dip each ball into the batter until well coated. Lay them out on two baking trays so they have plenty of space around them, and bake in the oven for 10 minutes. Then flip them over and bake for a further 10 minutes.

Polish Potato Pancakes with Cannellini Beans (*Placki Ziemniaczane*) ♡ ◉ ⊘

Steve's wife, Justyna, is from central Poland, and they often enjoy some *placki ziemniaczane* – here we bake them instead of frying them, to make them lighter and lower in calories, and we use cannellini beans to give them a little more character.

Serves 4 (makes about 10 small potato cakes)

Takes 35 minutes

3 tablespoons ground flax seeds
9 tablespoons water
5 medium potatoes (600g)
1 medium onion
1 x 400g tin of cannellini beans (approx. 240g when drained)
15g fresh chives
1 teaspoon salt
¼ teaspoon ground black pepper
½ teaspoon garlic powder
30g gram flour or buckwheat flour (use white flour as an alternative, or gluten-free if coeliac)

Preheat the oven to 200°C fan/220°C.

Put the ground flax seeds into a bowl with the water and set aside for 5 minutes.

Grate the potatoes, using a box grater or a food processor with the grater attachment. Peel and grate the onion separately and squeeze any excess liquid out.

Drain and rinse the cannellini beans, then put into a bowl and mash slightly. Using scissors, cut the chives into very small pieces.

Put all the ingredients into a large mixing bowl and mix well, using a spoon or by hand – the mixture will be slightly wet but the flour and flax seeds will hold it together.

Shape into small flat 6–7cm pancakes (75g each). Place them on two baking trays, lined with baking parchment to prevent them sticking to the tray, and bake in the preheated oven for 15 minutes. Then flip them over and bake for a further 10 minutes.

Serve with your favourite sauce – for example, see pages 186–7.

Celeriac Bhajis ♡ ✋ ⃠

A bhaji is the Indian version of a fritter, often coated with gram flour and seasoned with lots of different spices, then fried. The one that's most generally known in the West is the onion bhaji, but most veg make wonderful bhajis – here we use celeriac, but you can easily replace this with cauliflower or squash or pumpkin to make your own variation.

Makes 8 x 80g bhajis
Takes 30 minutes

1 large red onion
¼ celeriac (approx. 200g), or other veg of your preference
150g gram flour
¾ teaspoon baking powder
1 tablespoon ground cumin
1 tablespoon ground coriander
½ teaspoon ground chilli
1½ teaspoons salt
1 teaspoon ground turmeric

Preheat the oven to 200°C fan/220°C.

Peel the onion and cut it into long thin strips. Peel and grate the celeriac.

Pour 100ml of water into a large bowl. Sieve in the gram flour, baking powder, cumin, coriander, chilli, salt and turmeric and mix well. Mix in the onion and grated celeriac.

Divide the batter into 8 small burger shapes and lay them out on a large baking tray, lined with baking parchment to avoid sticking, and ensuring they each have enough space to bake.

Cook for 15 minutes in the preheated oven, then take out, turn the bhajis so they cook on both sides, put back and cook for a further 10 minutes.

Serve with your favourite sauce (see pages 186–7), or just on their own, or simply with hummus (see page 256).

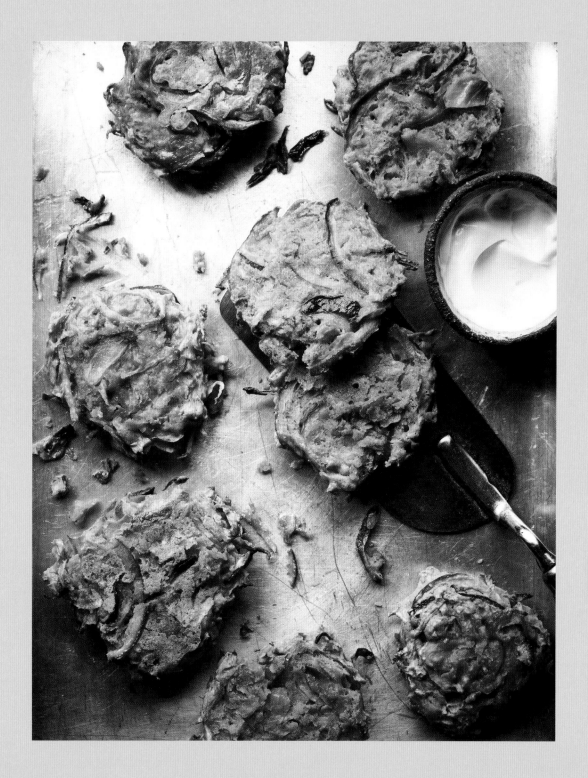

Toasted Wholemeal Pitta with Hummus, Rocket and Tomato ♡ ⓦ ◐ ⊜

This is so simple but at the same time very satisfying, and makes a great healthy lunch or snack at any time of day. It's a good option for anyone who is implementing a low-FODMAP diet. Below we give a basic recipe and a few suggestions to take your pitta to the next level.

Serves 1
Takes 5 minutes

1 gluten-free wholemeal pitta
    bread
½ a ripe tomato
a pinch of salt
50g low-FODMAP hummus
    (see page 256)
a handful of rocket

Suggested extras
30g cucumber
miso (a small amount, as it's
    very strong)
pickled red onions (see
    page 180)
20g sauerkraut
pitted Kalamata olives

Toast the wholemeal pitta until it's nice and crispy. Cut the tomato into thin slices and sprinkle it with a pinch of salt. Cut the pitta open and add a generous serving of hummus, some rocket and the tomato. Simple and tasty!

Grilled Veggie and Tofu Kebabs with Chimichurri Sauce ♡ ⊛ ◌ ⊜

Argentina is famous for mastering the art of cooking over an open flame, so it is no wonder their traditional chimichurri sauce with lots of fresh parsley, coriander and chilli goes perfectly with anything grilled.

Serves 4 (2 kebabs each)
Takes 30 minutes

Kebabs
150g oyster mushrooms
200g firm tofu
1 clove of garlic
4 tablespoons tamari/
    soy sauce (make sure to
    use gf soy sauce if you
    need to avoid gluten)
½ baguette or bread,
    preferably day-old (150g)
1 medium courgette
1 red onion
1 red pepper
8–10 cherry tomatoes

Chimichurri sauce
1 shallot
1 clove of garlic
25g fresh flat-leaf parsley
1 teaspoon fresh or dried
    oregano
½ teaspoon chilli flakes
3 tablespoons water
1 teaspoon red or white
    wine vinegar
juice of 1 lemon
salt and ground black pepper

Preheat the oven to 200°C fan/220°C.

If your skewers are wooden, soak them in water for 5 minutes – this will prevent them burning when you grill the kebabs. Easiest way to do this is to fill a 1 litre bottle with water, put the skewers in, and put the lid on.

Cut the oyster mushrooms into long strips. Cut the tofu into 8 even squares. Peel and finely chop the garlic. Put the tofu and mushrooms into a bowl, add the tamari/soy sauce and the chopped garlic, coat well and set aside until you are ready to assemble the kebabs.

While they are marinating, make the chimichurri sauce. Peel and finely chop the shallot, garlic, parsley and oregano, then put them all into a bowl with the rest of the sauce ingredients and mix well. Season with salt and ground black pepper to taste.

Trim the crusts off the bread and cut the bread into cubes roughly the same size as the tofu. Put them into a bowl and add 4 tablespoons of the chimichurri sauce, coating them well.

Cut the courgette into cubes a similar size to the tofu and bread. Peel the red onion, cut into quarters, then cut each of these quarters in half. Make sure you keep the pieces intact so they will fit on to the skewer. Cut the red pepper in half, removing the seeds, then cut into squares the width of the tofu. Put the courgettes, onions and peppers on a baking tray and bake in the preheated oven for 15 minutes.

Now it's time to skewer the kebabs. Start with an onion, then in any order you like add the cherry tomatoes, tofu, mushrooms, courgettes, bread cubes and peppers.

Cook on a high to medium heat on a griddle or in a non-stick pan, or ideally on the barbecue, for 3–4 minutes each side, until all the ingredients are cooked. They may need longer than 4 minutes. The thing to watch for is that the courgettes start to brown and char slightly – when that happens, turn and repeat with the next side.

Serve immediately, with a nice drizzle of the chimichurri sauce.

Veggie Pot Noodle with Miso   ⊘

The beauty of these is that you can prepare them, take them to work, then simply add boiling water, leave for 15 minutes and lunch is ready! If you can take some toasted sesame seeds or pickled ginger with you it will give you another element of flavour. These are quick to make and really deliver on flavour.

Serves 1
Takes 20 minutes

10g carrot
2 spring onions/scallions
¼ of a fresh red chilli
50g wholemeal noodles or
 brown rice noodles
½ teaspoon veg
 stock powder
1½ teaspoons miso
1 teaspoon curry powder
1 teaspoon fresh ginger
25g frozen peas
25g baby spinach
zest and juice of ½ a lime
1 teaspoon tamari/soy sauce
 (make sure to use gf soy
 sauce if you need to
 avoid gluten)

To serve
toasted sesame seeds
pickled ginger

Finely grate the carrot and slice the spring onions/scallions. Finely dice the red chilli (include the seeds if you like it spicy, or leave them out if you prefer it milder). Peel and grate the fresh ginger. Put the noodles into a large jar, along with the veg stock, miso and the rest of the ingredients.

When you are ready to eat, fill and boil a kettle. Once boiled, pour boiling water into the jar until everything is covered and leave it to sit for 15 minutes.

Serve with toasted sesame seeds and pickled ginger.

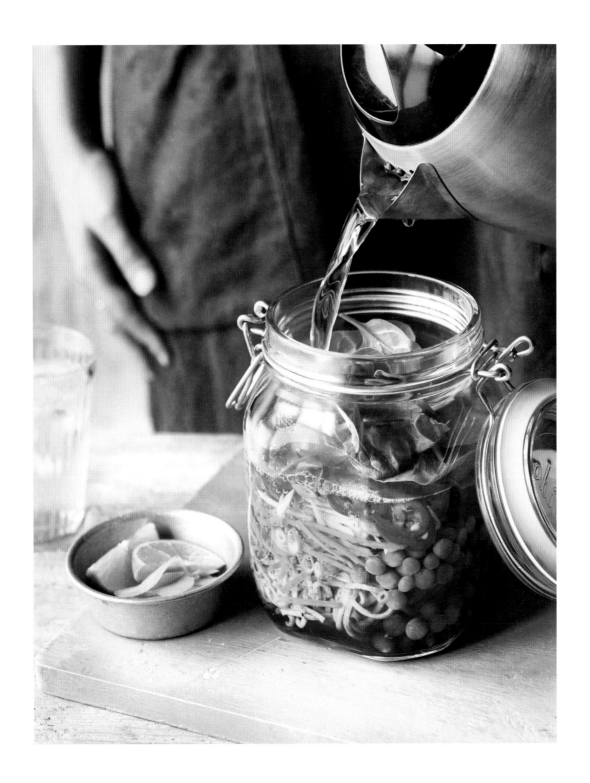

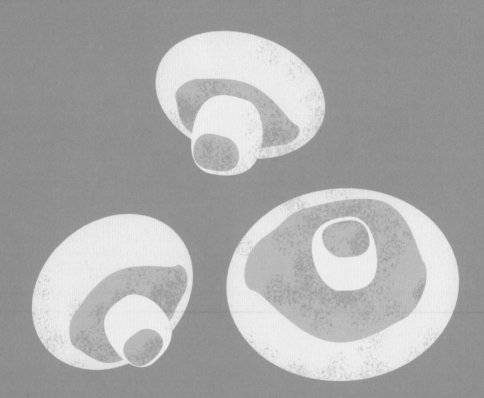

Chapter 12

Quick Easier Dinners

We excel at quick easy dinners, so we really hope you can adopt a dish or two from this section as part of your week. The time in which you can cook these will be improved by speedy knife skills and cooking on gas or induction, compared to electric. If you are on electric, make sure to give your oven and hob time to warm up before you get going.

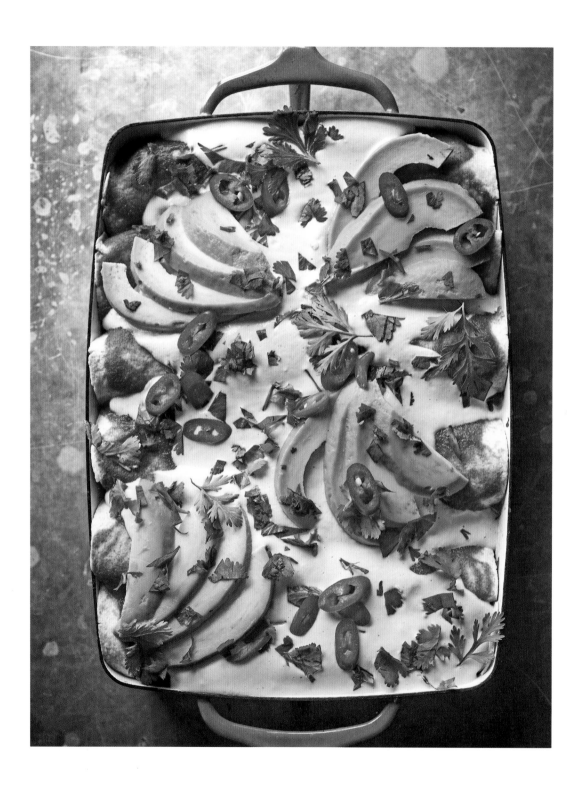

Easy Mexican Enchiladas ♡ ◯

The word enchilada comes from the Spanish word *enchilar*, which means to add chilli. Here, tortillas are filled with a delicious tomato and bean sauce, then baked in the oven and served with a rocking cashew cream – this is a family favourite in our house.

Serves 4–6
Takes 10–15 minutes

Cashew cream
100g cashew nuts
juice of ½ a lime
12 tablespoons non-dairy milk
½ teaspoon salt
a pinch of ground black pepper

Enchilada sauce
½ tablespoon chilli powder
1 teaspoon garlic powder
1 teaspoon ground cumin
½ teaspoon onion powder
200ml tomato purée
200ml veg stock
juice of ½ a lime
½ teaspoon salt
1 tablespoon maple syrup

Filling
1 x 400g tin of black beans (approx. 240g when drained)
1 x 200g tin of sweetcorn
1 x 400g jar of roasted red peppers in brine
6 medium wholemeal/corn tortillas

Garnish
a handful of fresh coriander (15g)
1 avocado
1 fresh red chilli

Preheat the oven to 250°C fan or the highest temperature your oven can go to if under 250°C. Put the cashew nuts into a bowl, cover with boiling water and leave to soak.

Put all the ingredients for the enchilada sauce into a bowl and whisk until smooth. Pour half of this mixture into a large bowl and set the other half to one side. Drain and rinse the black beans, sweetcorn and roasted red peppers. Chop the red peppers into thin strips. Add the beans, sweetcorn and red peppers to the large bowl of enchilada sauce and mix well.

Lay the tortillas out on a work surface one at a time, and fill them with the mixture, dividing it equally between the tortillas. Roll them up, then put them into an ovenproof dish or baking tray about 30cm x 20cm – 6 filled tortillas should fit perfectly. Once rolled, pour over the rest of the enchilada sauce and bake in the preheated oven for 5 minutes.

While the enchiladas are in the oven, drain and rinse the soaked cashew nuts. Put them into a blender with the rest of the ingredients for the cashew cream, and blend until smooth.

Finely chop the coriander stalks and leaves. Peel and slice the avocado, and finely slice the red chilli. Remove the enchiladas from the oven, drizzle over the cashew cream, and decorate with the sliced avocado, chilli and coriander.

Creamy Spiced Black Bean Quesadillas ♡ ✋ ⊘

Creamy, spicy, crispy and oh-so-delicious! These are low in fat, oil-free and take only 10–15 minutes to make – they are a wonderful dinner or healthy snack. Although tamari is not technically a Mexican condiment, it does give flavour and saves time, so it's worth using it if you can.

Makes 4 quesadillas
Takes 10–15 minutes

1 red onion
2 spring onions/scallions
10 cherry tomatoes
a small bunch of fresh coriander
1 fresh red chilli
1 avocado
1 x 400g tin of black beans (approx. 240g when drained)
1 teaspoon cumin seeds
1 teaspoon ground cumin
¼ teaspoon smoked paprika
¼ teaspoon ground cinnamon
¼ teaspoon ground black pepper
1 teaspoon ground coriander
1 tablespoon tamari/ soy sauce (make sure to use gf soy sauce if you need to avoid gluten)
juice of ½ lemon or 1 lime
a pinch of salt
4 wholewheat or corn tortillas

Cashew cheese
200g cashew nuts
150ml oat milk
½ teaspoon garlic powder
1 teaspoon lemon juice
½ teaspoon salt

Put the cashew nuts into a bowl, cover with boiling water and leave to soak for 5 minutes.

Peel the red onion and cut into thin strips. Slice the spring onions/scallions finely at an angle. Quarter the cherry tomatoes, and finely chop the coriander and red chilli (remove the seeds if you like it less spicy). Peel the avocado and cut into thin slices. Drain and rinse the black beans.

Heat a non-stick pan on a high heat. Once hot, add the onion, spring onions/scallions and chilli and cook for 2 minutes, stirring continuously. Add the spices, tamari/soy sauce, lemon or lime juice and salt, then cook for 30 seconds. Next add the drained beans and the cherry tomatoes and cook for 2 minutes, mashing and stirring. Set this filling aside.

Drain and rinse the cashew nuts. Put them into a blender along with the rest of the ingredients for the cashew cheese, and blend until super-smooth.

Clean the pan and dry it, put it on medium heat, and once hot add a tortilla and leave it to heat up for 10 seconds. Spoon on a generous serving of the cashew cheese (about 3 tablespoons per quesadilla) across the full tortilla. Add a good dollop of the fried black bean salsa to half the tortilla, and top with sliced avocado, chopped coriander and a sprinkle of chilli. Fold over the tortilla, and once it's starting to brown and crisp up around the corners, remove from the pan and slice into quarters on a chopping board. Repeat with the remaining tortillas and fillings.

Keep any remaining cashew cheese to use for other sandwiches – it will last for 5 days in the fridge.

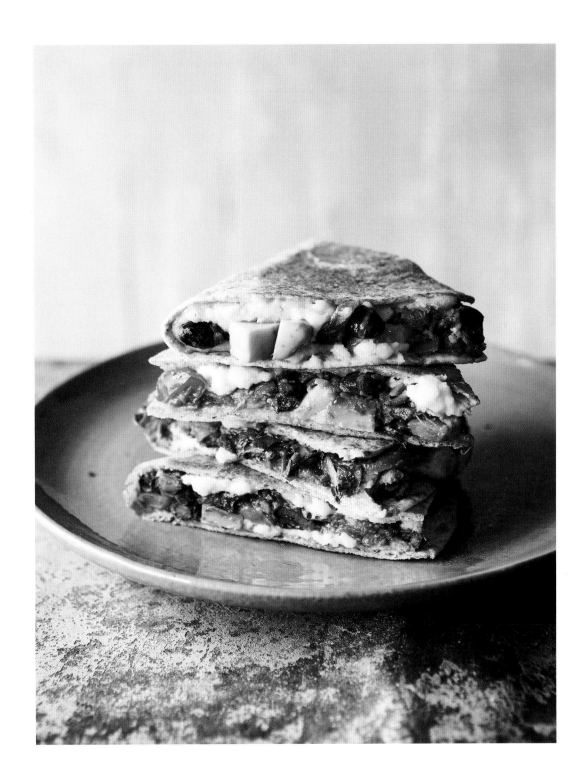

Easy Light Spicy Tacos ♡ ✋ ⊘

These are quick, delicious and make a wonderful summer dinner, lunch or snack. Tacos are the ultimate street food, in that they are filling, are made to be hand-sized, are super-customizable to your taste and are packed full of flavour. Here we use baby gem lettuce leaves instead of tortillas, as they're lighter, crunchier and super-quick to make, but you can easily use wholemeal or corn tortillas if you prefer. We make a lovely spicy jackfruit filling and add some sauerkraut and avocado to give you a delicious creamy and acidic crunch.

Serves 2–4
Takes 15 minutes

1 x 400g tin of jackfruit
1 avocado
2 baby gem lettuces
100g sauerkraut (red sauerkraut looks better if you can get it)

Dressing
2 tablespoons tomato purée
2 tablespoons tamari/ soy sauce (make sure to use gf soy sauce if you need to avoid gluten)
2 tablespoons maple syrup
1 teaspoon apple cider vinegar
1 teaspoon smoked paprika
1 teaspoon ground cumin
½ teaspoon chilli powder
½ teaspoon garlic powder/ granules

To garnish
1 fresh red chilli
2 spring onions/scallions

Drain and rinse the jackfruit and cut it into thin strips. In a bowl mix together the dressing ingredients.

Heat a large non-stick frying pan on a high heat. Once hot, add the jackfruit and fry for 4–5 minutes, stirring occasionally, until it starts to brown slightly. Add the dressing to the pan and mix well, ensuring it is all well coated. Cook for 2 minutes, then remove and set aside.

Cut the avocado into quarters, remove the stone and skin, and slice the flesh into thin strips. Finely slice the chilli and spring onions/scallions for the garnish.

To make your taco shells, remove the outer layers of the baby gem lettuce – you should get 4 or 5 large leaves per baby gem. Lay them out on a board and divide the jackfruit between them. Add a slice of avocado to each one, and a nice amount of sauerkraut.

Garnish with some sliced chilli and spring onions/scallions and enjoy!

If you want to make these spicier, add some of our homemade sriracha sauce (see page 187).

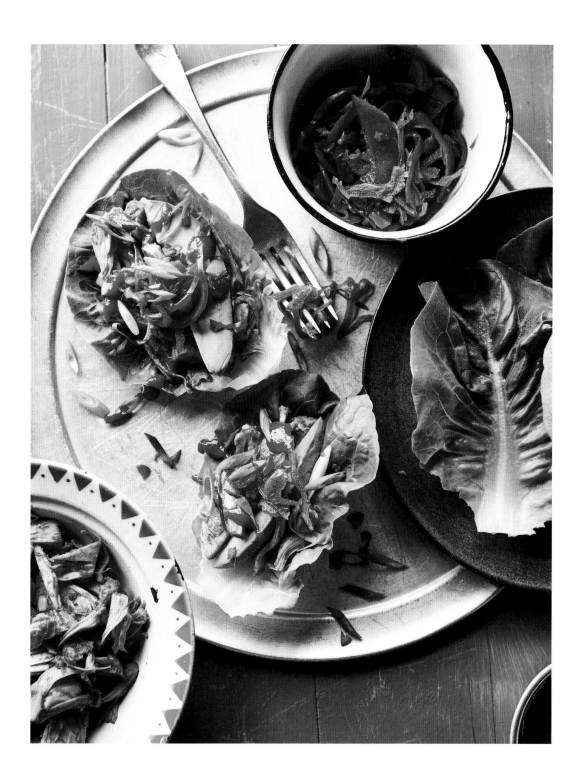

Pan-fried Tofu with Steamed Greens and Quinoa ♡ ✋ ⊘ ⊜

A lovely, simple dinner that is really nourishing and wholesome. This is one of our good friend Mark Lawlor's staple dinners, which we have eaten on many a mid-week night around his stove.

Serves 4
Takes 20 minutes

200g spinach/kale/chard/
  green cabbage
2 x 450g blocks of firm tofu
2½cm cube of fresh ginger
  (15g)
1 fresh red chilli
200g fresh tomatoes
30g sesame seeds
5 tablespoons tamari/
  soy sauce (make sure to
  use gf soy sauce if you
  need to avoid gluten)
1 tablespoon maple syrup
juice of 1 lime
400g pre-cooked quinoa or
  brown rice

To serve
80g sauerkraut

Wash your greens, roughly chop them into small bite-size pieces, then put them into a steamer (or you could use a colander over a pan of water) and steam for 3 minutes, or until they are soft but not overcooked. You will have to turn them once or twice, to ensure they all cook evenly. Set aside.

Cut the tofu into ½cm cubes. Peel the ginger and deseed the chilli – you can leave the seeds in if you like it hot – then finely chop them. Cut the tomatoes into bite-size pieces.

Put a medium-sized non-stick pan on a high heat. Once hot, add the ginger and chilli and fry on a high heat for 2 minutes, then remove from the pan. Add the tofu and sesame seeds and fry for a further 5 minutes, stirring regularly until they start to brown on each side.

Mix together the tamari/soy sauce and maple syrup and add to the pan (it should make a loud hissing sound). Quickly move them around the pan, allowing the tamari/soy sauce to reduce and coat all the tofu. Add your steamed greens, along with the tomatoes, fried ginger and chilli and the lime juice. Mix through, then cook for a further 3–4 minutes, continuing to stir regularly.

Heat the pre-cooked quinoa or brown rice according to the packet instructions.

Ideally, serve this all together in a bowl, with the quinoa/rice on the bottom and the tofu, greens and sesame mix on the top. Garnish with a generous amount of sauerkraut per portion.

Serving suggestion: sprinkle some nutritional yeast on top for a cheesy flavour.

Teriyaki Noodles ♡ ⊛ ◌ ⊜

This is our take on teriyaki noodles. It's a tasty and quick dinner that is really flavoursome and easy to make. We use buckwheat or brown rice noodles.

Serves 3
Takes 15 minutes

150g buckwheat noodles/
　　brown rice noodles
a thumb-size piece of
　　fresh ginger
a handful of spring onions/
　　scallions (green part only)
½ a fresh red chilli
150g oyster mushrooms
1 red pepper
1 head of pak choi
　　(225g max)
4 tablespoons tamari/
　　soy sauce (make sure to
　　use gf soy sauce if you
　　need to avoid gluten)
1 tablespoon maple syrup
juice of 2 limes

Garnish
chilli flakes
10g toasted sesame seeds
fresh coriander

Bring a small pot of water to the boil and cook the noodles according to the packet instructions, then drain and rinse them in cold water so they don't stick together. Set aside.

Peel and finely chop the ginger. Finely slice the spring onions/scallions, and finely chop the chilli, removing the seeds if you don't like it spicy. Chop the mushrooms up nice and small, then deseed the red pepper and finely chop it, along with the pak choi.

Heat a wok or a large non-stick frying pan on a high heat. Once the pan is hot, add the ginger, chilli, spring onions/scallions and red pepper and cook for 2 minutes, stirring regularly. Then add the mushrooms and cook for another 3 minutes, stirring regularly – if they start to stick, add a teaspoon of water and stir to loosen.

While these are cooking, prepare your sauce by mixing the tamari/soy sauce, maple syrup and lime juice together in a bowl. Add half the sauce to the pan along with the pak choi and cook for 2 minutes.

Add the drained noodles, together with the remaining sauce, and cook for a further 2–3 minutes. Chop the coriander for the garnish.

Remove from the heat and serve, topped with chilli flakes, toasted sesame seeds and chopped coriander.

Japanese Veg and Noodle Ramen ♡ ✋ ⊘ ⊜

Ramen is one of the most popular dishes in Japan. It's fresh-tasting and simple to whip up. We designed this dish to be really easy to make, using ingredients that you can get anywhere. It's perfect for a nourishing mid-week dinner.

Serves 4
Takes 10–15 minutes

2 litres veg stock (garlic- and onion-free)
5½ tablespoons tamari/soy sauce (make sure to use gf soy sauce if you need to avoid gluten)
a thumb-size piece of fresh ginger, grated
juice of 2 limes
2 tablespoons maple syrup
300g oyster mushrooms
3 tablespoons water
4 nests of brown rice noodles (200g)

Toppings
1 fresh red chilli
4 spring onions/scallions (green parts only)
1 large carrot
1 x 200g pack of beansprouts

To garnish
sauerkraut (20g per person to be low-FODMAP)
sesame seeds

To prepare the broth, first put the veg stock into a large non-stick pan with 2½ tablespoons of tamari/soy sauce, the grated ginger, the juice of 1 lime and 1 tablespoon of maple syrup, and bring to the boil.

Tear or chop the mushrooms into bite-size pieces. Put a pan on a high heat, and once hot, add the mushrooms and cook for 2–3 minutes, stirring regularly (if they start to stick, add a teaspoon of water and stir to loosen them).

Mix the remaining 3 tablespoons of tamari/soy sauce, the 3 tablespoons of water, the juice of the second lime and the remaining tablespoon of maple syrup together in a bowl and add to the mushrooms. Cook for 2 minutes, or until most of the sauce has been absorbed.

Once your broth is boiling, reduce to a simmer, then add the noodles and cook according to the packet instructions.

In the meantime, start preparing the toppings: deseed and finely chop the red chilli, together with the green part of the spring onions/scallions. Grate the carrot and rinse the beansprouts.

Once the noodles are cooked, divide them between four deep bowls, spooning them out of the pan with a slotted spoon or tongs. Ladle out the broth and put equal amounts into each bowl, so that the noodles are just covered.

Now, layer your ramen with the toppings: beansprouts and grated carrot on either side of each bowl, with the chopped spring onions/scallions and chilli in the centre.

Finally, add the mushrooms and sauerkraut right in the middle, sprinkle with sesame seeds and serve.

Top tip: to take your ramen to the next level, add some dried seaweed (e.g. arami) and 2 tablespoons of miso to your broth, and add fresh coriander and/or pickled ginger to the garnish.

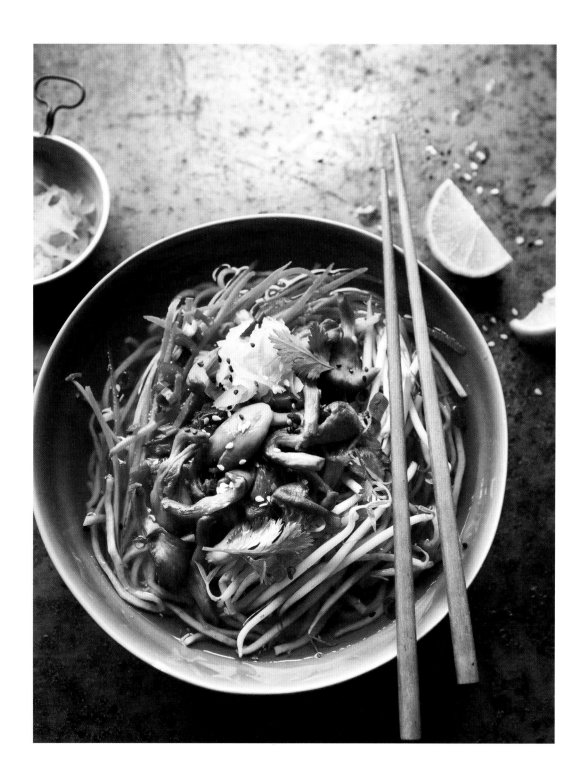

Quick Burger ♡ ✋ ◌ ☺

This recipe came out of our 'feburgruary' series, where for the month of February we filmed nothing but burger recipes on our YouTube channel! To make this burger gut-friendly, use a gluten-free bun or a baby gem lettuce slider.

Serves 6 (makes 6 x 115g burgers)
Takes 15 minutes (longer if cooking your own quinoa)

180g cooked quinoa (store-bought pre-cooked, or cook your own – see method)
210g drained tinned chickpeas
2 large leeks, green parts only (200g)
½ a thumb-size piece of fresh ginger
1 fresh red chilli
100g oyster mushrooms
2 tablespoons tamari/soy sauce (make sure to use gf soy sauce if you need to avoid gluten)
1 teaspoon balsamic vinegar
1 teaspoon salt
½ teaspoon ground black pepper
2 tablespoons nutritional yeast

Binder

3 tablespoons ground flax seeds
9 tablespoons water
4 tablespoons rice flour

To serve

gluten-free burger buns
lettuce
mustard
gherkins
tomatoes
low-FODMAP hummus (see page 256)

Boil a kettle and cook the quinoa (90–100g uncooked) following the packet instructions, then allow to cool, or simply use store-bought pre-cooked quinoa. Rinse the chickpeas.

To make your flax egg, mix the ground flax seeds and water in a bowl and set aside for 5 minutes, or until you are ready to make the burgers.

Cut the leek greens into very thin semi-circles. Rinse thoroughly in a colander to remove all the sediment, then drain. Peel and chop the ginger finely, deseed the chilli, and cut the oyster mushrooms into small bite-size pieces.

Put a medium-sized non-stick pan on a high heat, then add the leek greens, ginger and chilli and reduce the heat to medium, stirring for 4–5 minutes until the greens reduce. If they start to stick, add a teaspoon of water and stir to loosen.

Add the mushrooms and cook for a minute, then add the tamari/soy sauce, coating all the veg well, and cook for another 2–3 minutes. Remove from the heat and allow to cool.

Put the chickpeas into a bowl and mash them, using a fork. Add the cooked quinoa, the mushroom and ginger mixture, the vinegar, salt, pepper, nutritional yeast and the flax egg. Mix well, then add the rice flour and stir until incorporated. If you prefer a smoother, more homogeneous burger, blend the ingredients in a food processor until nice and smooth. Now shape into 5 or 6 burgers.

Clean out the pan and add 1 teaspoon of oil, then, using kitchen paper, spread the oil around the pan and remove the paper so that you have the tiniest coating of oil possible. Bring to a medium heat and add 2 or 3 burgers at a time. Cook for 2–3 minutes on each side, until golden brown and heated through.

Serve in gluten-free buns or lettuce cups, with mustard, gherkins, tomatoes and our low-FODMAP hummus.

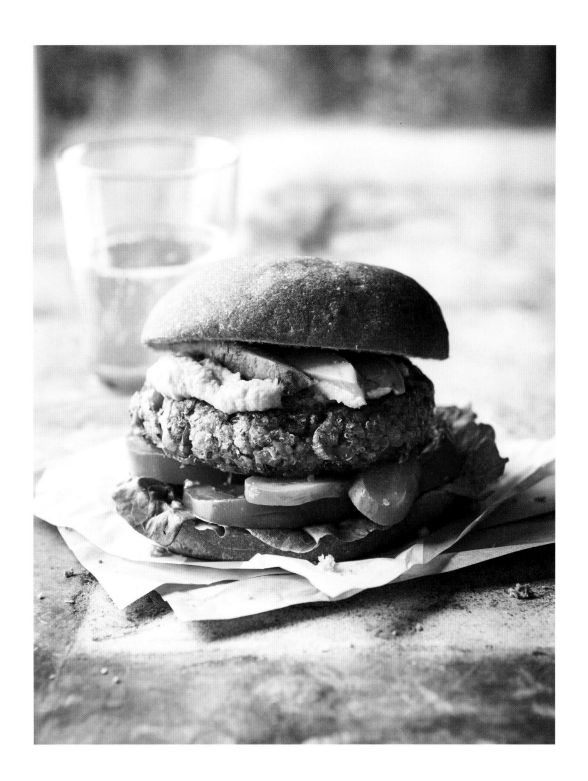

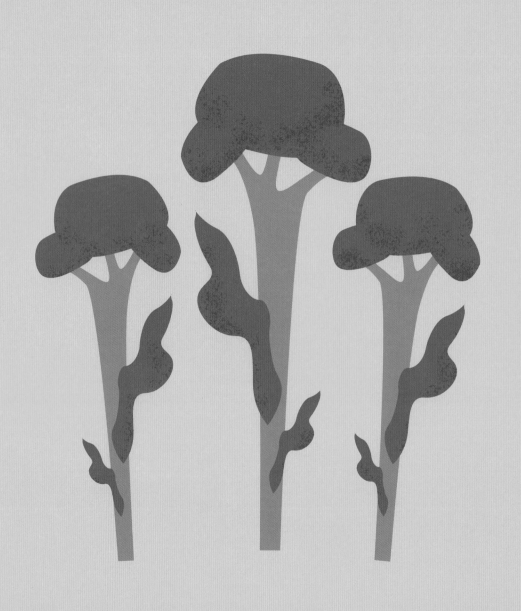

Chapter 13

One Pot Dinners

As the name implies, there is less of a clean-up with these dinners. They work great as part of a meal prep, and serve well cold as a lunch the next day.

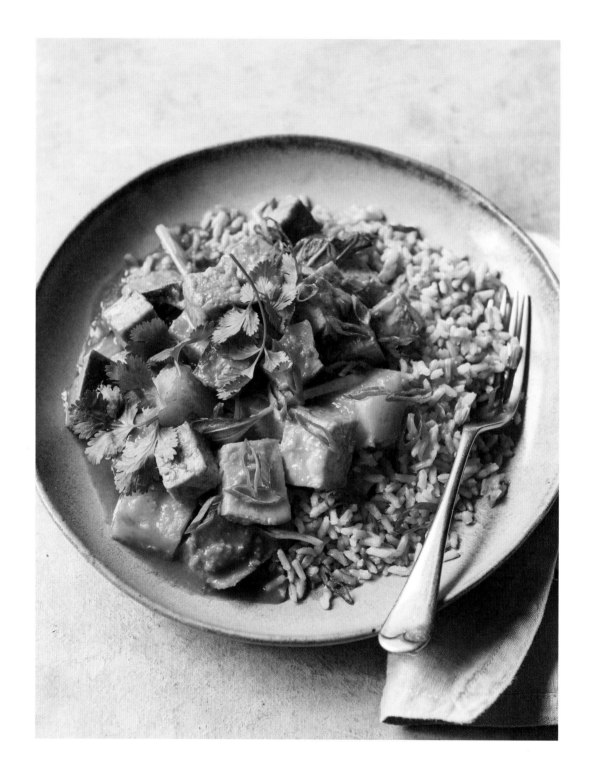

Vietnamese Coconut and Tempeh Curry ♡ ⚝ ◌ ⊜

This is a deliciously simple curry! Tempeh is a fermented soy bean block, originally from Indonesia. We know it's not a very appealing description, but when prepared right, this dish is packed with flavour and really filling. Tempeh is not as readily available as tofu, but it can be found in most good health stores. If you can't find it, just replace it with tofu. We like to serve this curry with short-grain brown rice.

Serves 4
Takes 35 minutes

300g sweet potatoes
400g potatoes
1 teaspoon salt
a thumb-size piece of
  fresh ginger
220ml full-fat coconut milk
400ml water
juice of 2 limes
2 tablespoons maple syrup
2 tablespoons curry powder
4 tablespoons tamari/
  soy sauce (make sure to
  use gf soy sauce if you
  need to avoid gluten)
1 x 300g pack of tempeh (if
  not available, substitute
  firm tofu/oyster
  mushrooms)
½ a head of pak choi
ground black pepper

To serve
a small bunch of spring
  onions/scallions (green
  part only)
a bunch of fresh coriander

Preheat the oven to 180°C fan/200°C.

Chop the sweet potatoes and regular potatoes into bite-size pieces (leaving the skin on). Put on a baking tray with a generous pinch of salt, mix well and bake in the preheated oven for 25 minutes. Peel and finely dice the ginger.

To make the dressing, put the coconut milk, water, ginger, lime juice, maple syrup, curry powder and tamari/soy sauce into a blender, and whiz until smooth.

Cut the tempeh/tofu into small cubes (around 1½cm) – the smaller they are, the more flavour each piece will have. Put on a baking tray and dress with about half the dressing. It's important to mix the tempeh and the sauce well, to make sure each piece is full of flavour, and also to make sure that the tempeh is well spread out on the baking tray. Put into the oven alongside the potatoes and bake for 20 minutes. After 10 minutes, stir the tempeh to ensure that the dressing is well distributed.

Meanwhile, pour the other half of the dressing into a large pan – this will become the sauce for the dish, along with any remaining sauce from the baked tempeh. Bring to the boil, then lower the heat and reduce to a simmer.

Once the tempeh and potatoes are done, transfer them into the pan of simmering sauce and mix well. Finely chop the pak choi, removing the nub at the end, and add to the pan.

Remove from the heat, taste and season. Finely slice the spring onions/scallions (make sure you just use the green tops) and fresh coriander, and sprinkle them over the dish when serving.

Low-FODMAP Malaysian Laksa Curry ♡ ✋ ◌ ⊜

This is rich, sweet, savoury and delicious, and it takes only 10 minutes to make. We came up with this recipe when our friend Dr Rupy came round to shoot a recipe video. His mom is from Malaysia and he didn't believe we could cook a laksa curry in 5 minutes that would taste as good as hers – we did just that, and here's the delicious recipe. We adjusted that original recipe to be low-FODMAP and also gave it an extra 5 minutes, so you could take your time and enjoy it more.

Serves 4
Takes 10 minutes

4 nests of brown rice noodles/ buckwheat noodles (200g)

The paste
a thumb-size piece of fresh ginger
1 fresh red chilli
1 tablespoon ground turmeric
juice of 1 lime
1 tablespoon maple syrup
1 tablespoon coriander seeds
1 tablespoon cumin seeds
240ml full-fat coconut milk
160ml water
2 tablespoons tamari/soy sauce (make sure to use gf soy sauce if you need to avoid gluten)

The rest
150g tofu/tempeh
2 tablespoons tamari/soy sauce (make sure to use gf soy sauce if you need to avoid gluten)
1 carrot
½ a courgette
salt

fresh coriander/ basil leaves
juice of 1 lime
fresh red chillies

Fill and boil a kettle. Pour boiling water into a saucepan and add the noodles. Cook according to the packet instructions, then drain and put them into cold water so they don't stick together.

Peel the ginger and roughly slice the chilli lengthwise, including the seeds if you like it hot and omitting them if you prefer it milder.

Put all the paste ingredients into a blender and blend until smooth. Grate the carrot and courgette. Finely chop the tofu/ tempeh into small bite-size pieces. Chop the coriander/basil and finely slice the red chillies for the garnish.

Heat a non-stick frying pan on a high heat. Once hot, add the tofu or tempeh and fry until brown on all sides – this should take 3–4 minutes. If it starts to stick, add a teaspoon of water and stir to loosen. Add the tamari/soy sauce and stir quickly, spreading it around to coat all the tofu/tempeh. Add the grated carrot and courgette and a generous pinch of salt and cook for 1–2 minutes. Add the paste and cook for another minute.

Using a slotted spoon, remove the noodles from the water and add them to the frying pan. Finally add the coriander/basil and the lime juice and heat for a few seconds. Garnish with finely sliced red chilli and enjoy!

Humble Lentil Stew with Raita ⊘ ✋ ⊘

This is a lovely chunky super-wholesome stew. You could speed up the cooking time by using tinned lentils, but dried lentils give a deeper, more substantial taste and the opportunity to layer on more flavour.

Serves 6
Takes 45 minutes

1 onion (250g)
3 cloves of garlic
1 beetroot (150g)
2 medium potatoes (500g)
2 carrots (250g)
2 medium leeks (300g)
1 teaspoon salt
½ teaspoon ground black pepper
1 teaspoon smoked paprika
1 x 400g tin of chopped tomatoes
150g dried Puy/ green/ brown lentils
4 tablespoons tamari/ soy sauce (make sure to use gf soy sauce if you need to avoid gluten)
2 bay leaves
20g kombu/dulse seaweed (optional)
4 sprigs of fresh thyme
1 small sprig of fresh rosemary
juice of ½ a lemon
2 litres veg stock or water
100g baby spinach

Raita
100g cucumber
200g coconut yoghurt or soy yoghurt
2 tablespoons maple syrup
2 teaspoons lime juice
a pinch of salt

Peel and finely slice the onion and garlic. Finely chop the beetroot, potatoes and carrots into small bite-size pieces. Cut the leeks in half lengthwise and give them a good clean inside, as sediment is often hiding there. Then cut them into small bite-size pieces.

Heat a large family-size pot (4 litres) on a high heat. Add the onion, carrot, leek, potatoes and beetroot, garlic, salt and black pepper. Fry for 5 minutes, stirring occasionally so nothing sticks, then cover with a lid, turn down the heat to medium, and sweat for 10 minutes, stirring occasionally. If it does start to stick, add a tablespoon of water and stir to loosen everything again – repeat if needed.

Add the smoked paprika, tomatoes, lentils, tamari/soy sauce, bay leaves, kombu/dulse (if using), the leaves from the sprigs of thyme and rosemary, the lemon juice and the veg stock, and turn up the heat to high. Stir a few times, bring to the boil, then reduce the heat to a simmer for 20 minutes, or until the lentils have cooked and the potato, beetroot and carrot are soft to the bite. Season with salt and pepper to your taste. Add the spinach before serving.

To make the raita, finely grate the cucumber and put it into a sieve to drain, then squeeze out any excess water. Put the yoghurt into a bowl and add the cucumber along with the maple syrup, lime juice and salt. Mix well.

To serve, put a generous serving of lentil stew into each bowl, with a lovely drizzle of raita on top – and enjoy this hearty bowl of loveliness!

Spinach and
Butter Bean Curry ♡ ⊛ ◌ ⊜

This is a simple and delicious butter bean curry that is quick to make. Garnish with sesame seeds for an extra pop of flavour. A perfect warming hug in a bowl for a cold day.

Serves 4
Takes 10–15 minutes

a thumb-size piece of
    fresh ginger
1 bunch of spring onions/
    scallions (green part only)
1 fresh red chilli
200g oyster mushrooms
100g green beans
150g broccoli
140g drained tinned
    butter beans
2 tablespoons tamari/
    soy sauce (make sure to
    use gf soy sauce if you
    need to avoid gluten)
100g baby spinach
1½ tablespoons curry powder
1 teaspoon ground cumin
160ml coconut milk
150ml water
1 x 400g tin of chopped
    tomatoes
juice of 1 lime
salt and ground black pepper

Peel and finely chop the ginger. Finely chop the green parts of the spring onions/scallions and the chilli (removing the seeds if you don't like it spicy). The white parts of the spring onions/scallions freeze well to use in another dish. Finely chop the oyster mushrooms, chop the green beans in half, and cut the broccoli into bite-size florets. Drain and rinse the butter beans.

Put a large non-stick pan on a high heat. Once hot, add the ginger, chilli and spring onions/scallions and cook for 1–2 minutes, stirring regularly.

Add the mushrooms, green beans and broccoli florets and cook for a further 3 minutes. Add 2 tablespoons of tamari/soy sauce and cook for a further minute, then add all the remaining ingredients and bring to the boil.

Once boiling, reduce to a simmer for 2–3 minutes, then remove from the heat. Taste to see if it needs any further seasoning, then serve.

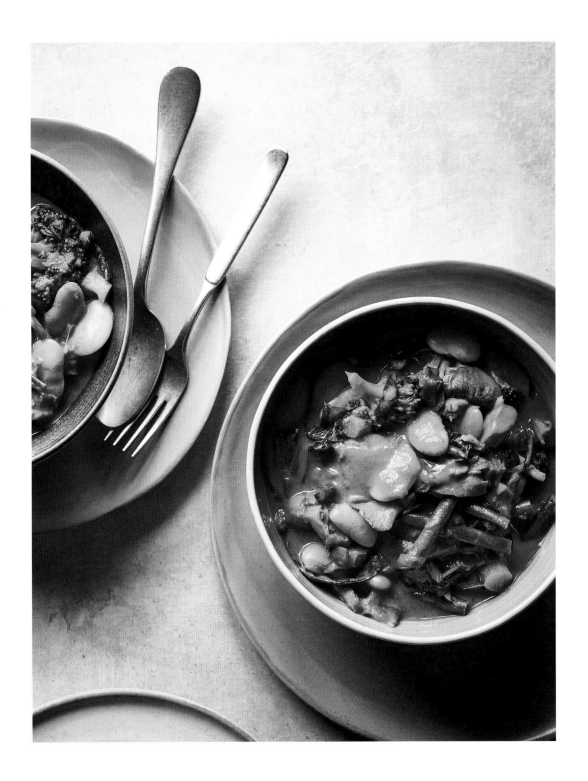

Jambalaya ♡ ✋ ⃠

This lovely stewed rice and veg dish comes from New Orleans, with roots in West Africa, France and Spain. Here we use the southern US holy trinity of base veg – onion, celery and green pepper – cooked with vegan sausage and spices to give it its typical 'meaty' bite, then add the rice and cook it with the veg to make a really delicious dinner or cold lunch the next day. We added a few more aromatic spices to give it an extra subtle sweet aroma.

Serves 4
Takes 50 minutes

1 medium onion
1 green pepper
3 stalks of celery
300g vegan sausages
½ teaspoon smoked paprika
2 tablespoons sweet paprika
1 teaspoon garlic powder
½ teaspoon ground
    black pepper
1 teaspoon dried oregano
½ teaspoon cayenne or
    chilli powder
a pinch of ground cloves
1 cinnamon stick
1½ teaspoons salt
200g brown basmati rice
800ml veg stock
3 sprigs of fresh thyme
juice of ½ a lemon
30g toasted cashew nuts,
    to serve

Peel and finely dice the onion, green pepper and celery. Cut the vegan sausages into bite-size pieces. Heat a large pan on a high heat, then add the onion, green pepper, celery and vegan sausages and fry for 10 minutes, stirring regularly to avoid them sticking. If they do start to stick, add a tablespoon of water and stir to loosen.

Once the onions have started to brown, add the smoked paprika, sweet paprika, garlic powder, black pepper, oregano, cayenne or chilli, cloves, cinnamon, salt and the uncooked rice, and cook for 1–2 minutes, stirring regularly.

Add the veg stock and the thyme leaves (removed from their stalks), and bring to the boil. Once boiling, reduce to a simmer, put the lid on and leave to cook for 30 minutes, until the rice is soft. Add the lemon juice, stir, taste and adjust the seasoning to your palate. Garnish with the toasted cashew nuts.

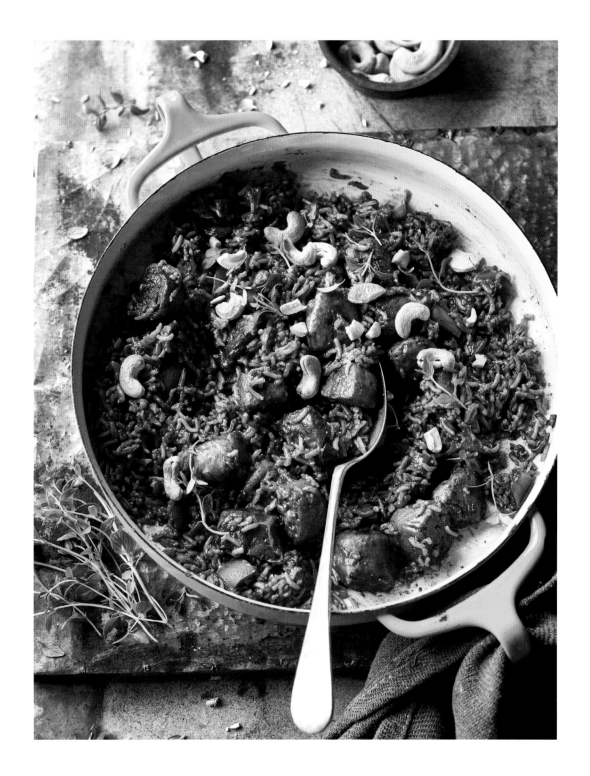

Next Level Chilli Sin Carne ♡ ✋ ⊘

The addition of almond butter and cocoa with a lot of aromatic spices really adds a depth that takes this chilli to another level.

Serves 4
Takes 45 minutes

1 red onion
4 cloves of garlic
250g oyster mushrooms
1 fresh green chilli
1 red pepper
1 yellow pepper
1 x 400g tin of black beans
    (approx. 240g when drained)
1 tablespoon cumin seeds/
    ground cumin
1 teaspoon coriander seeds/
    ground coriander
1 teaspoon sesame seeds
1 tablespoon tamari/soy sauce
    (make sure to use gf soy sauce
    if you need to avoid gluten)
1½ teaspoons salt
2 x 400g tins of chopped
    tomatoes
¼ teaspoon smoked paprika
2 tablespoons almond butter/
    peanut butter
2 tablespoons cocoa powder
1 cinnamon stick/1 teaspoon
    ground cinnamon
1 bay leaf
1 tablespoon maple syrup
¼ teaspoon ground black pepper
20g fresh coriander
juice of ½ a lime

Quick-fire coriander yoghurt
½ a bunch of fresh coriander
200g coconut/soy yoghurt
a pinch of salt
a pinch of ground black pepper
juice of 1 lime

Peel and finely dice the onion and garlic. Roughly chop the oyster mushrooms into bite-size pieces. Finely chop the green chilli (leaving the seeds in if you like it spicier). Chop the red and yellow peppers into small bite-size pieces. Drain and rinse the black beans.

Heat a large, wide-bottomed non-stick pan on a medium heat. Add the cumin, coriander and sesame seeds and toast for 4–5 minutes, stirring regularly, until the cumin seeds start to pop. Remove and grind to a powder in a pestle and mortar. If you don't have one, put the seeds into a ziplock bag, close it, and crush them using a rolling pin. Remove and set aside.

Turn the heat under the pan up to high and add the chopped oyster mushrooms. Using another pan that is slightly smaller, push it down on the mushrooms to compress them. This squeezes the water out of the mushrooms and encourages them to brown more and develop more flavour. Cook for about 3–4 minutes, compressing them, then turn the mushrooms over and repeat until they are nice and brown on both sides. Add the tamari/soy sauce and cook for 1 minute, stirring the mushrooms around well. Remove from the pan and set aside.

Add the chopped onion and chilli to the pan and cook for 4 minutes, stirring regularly. If they start to stick, add a teaspoon of water and stir to loosen them. Once they are starting to brown, add the garlic, the chopped peppers and a pinch of salt, and cook with the lid on for a further 4 minutes, stirring regularly.

Add the chopped tomatoes, smoked paprika, salt, black beans, almond butter, cocoa powder, cinnamon, bay leaf and maple syrup, along with the toasted spices, cooked mushrooms and black pepper. Turn up the heat to high until it starts to boil. Then reduce the heat and leave to simmer for a further 5 minutes. Finely chop the fresh coriander and add to the pan with the lime juice.

For the coriander yoghurt, finely chop the coriander and add to the yoghurt with the rest of the ingredients. Mix well and use to garnish your next level chilli.

Spicy African Peanut Stew ⊛ ⊘

This is a staple dish in western Africa, where they make a sauce with peanut paste and tomatoes, called *maafe*. Here we use oyster mushrooms to create a chewy bite along with the chickpeas – try to keep the strips of oyster mushroom long so that they are more prominent. There are some wonderful aromatic spices here to elevate this dish. It's quick, really tasty and deeply satisfying!

Serves 4
Takes 25 minutes

2 onions
2 cloves of garlic
½ a thumb-size piece
  of ginger
1 fresh red chilli (more if you
  like it spicy)
1 x 400g tin of chickpeas
  (approx. 240g when
  drained)
250g oyster mushrooms
2 sweet potatoes
¼ of a head of white
  cabbage (250g)
1½ teaspoons salt
450ml veg stock
1 tablespoon ground cumin
1 tablespoon ground
  coriander
1 tablespoon sweet paprika
125g peanut butter
1 x 400g tin of chopped
  tomatoes
100g baby spinach
juice of 1 lime

Peel and finely dice the onions, garlic and ginger. Finely slice the chilli, leaving the seeds in if you like it hotter and removing them if you want less heat. Drain and rinse the chickpeas and pull the oyster mushrooms into long thin strips, using your hands. Chop the sweet potatoes into small bite-size pieces, leaving the skin on (remove any bruises or less savoury bits). Cut the cabbage into long thin strips.

Heat a large, wide-bottomed non-stick pan on a high heat. Once hot, add the prepared onions, garlic, ginger, chilli and mushrooms and fry for 5–6 minutes, stirring regularly to prevent them sticking. If they do start to stick, add a teaspoon of water and stir to loosen.

Once the onions have started to brown, add the chopped sweet potatoes and cabbage, a pinch of salt and 50ml of veg stock. Stir, then put the lid on and allow to cook for 10–15 minutes, until the sweet potatoes start to soften, stirring occasionally. Remove the lid, add the ground cumin, coriander and paprika, and mix well.

Put the remaining veg stock and the peanut butter into a jug and mix so that it starts to combine (if the veg stock is still warm it makes it much easier to emulsify and mix well). Pour this sauce over the cooked veg, add the tomatoes, bring to the boil, then reduce to a simmer for 5 minutes. Add the baby spinach and the lime juice, then taste and adjust the seasoning with more salt, pepper and lime.

Southern Indian Sweet Potato and Lentil Curry ♡ ✋ ⊘

Southern Indian cooking often uses the creaminess of coconut combined with hot spices to give really balanced meals bursting with flavour. This curry is no exception, with sweet coconut and tangy tamarind giving a really rounded curry.

Serves 4
Takes 50 minutes

1 tablespoon cumin seeds/
  ground cumin
1 tablespoon coriander seeds/
  ground coriander
1 teaspoon mustard seeds
20g desiccated coconut
3 spring onions/scallions
2 cloves of garlic
3cm piece of fresh ginger
½ a fresh red chilli
1 medium sweet potato (300g)
1 red pepper
1 head of broccoli (approx. 250g)
1 aubergine
1 teaspoon salt
1 tablespoon curry powder
½ teaspoon ground black pepper
1 tablespoon tamari/soy sauce
  (use gf soy sauce if you
  avoid gluten)
2 litres veg stock or water
1 x 400ml tin of low-fat
  coconut milk
200g split red lentils
1 tablespoon tamarind pulp, or
  ½ tablespoon lime juice +
  ½ tablespoon coconut sugar/
  brown sugar
10g fresh coriander/
  flat-leaf parsley
100g baby spinach

To garnish
pickled ginger

Heat a large pot on a high heat. Add the cumin seeds, coriander seeds, mustard seeds and desiccated coconut and toast for 3–4 minutes, until the cumin seeds start to pop. Remove from the pot, grind in a pestle and mortar until smooth. If you don't have one, leave them to cool, then put them into a ziplock bag, seal and use a rolling pin to gently bash them to a powder.

Peel and roughly chop the spring onions/scallions, garlic and ginger. Dice the chilli, including the seeds if you like it hot. Chop the sweet potato, red pepper, broccoli and aubergine into small bite-size pieces so that they will cook quickly.

Put the same large pot back on a high heat. Once hot, add the spring onions/scallions and fry on a high heat for 4 minutes, stirring continuously. If they start to stick, add ½ teaspoon of water and stir to loosen. Add the chopped garlic, ginger and chilli and fry for 2 minutes: the spring onions/scallions should be starting to brown and the garlic should be going golden.

Add the chopped broccoli, sweet potato, aubergine and pepper, together with the salt, curry powder, toasted ground spices and toasted coconut, ground black pepper and tamari/soy sauce. Add 50ml of the veg stock and mix well. Put the lid on the pot, turn the heat down to medium and leave to cook for 10 minutes, stirring occasionally.

Add the coconut milk, lentils, the remaining veg stock or water and the tamarind pulp and stir well. Turn the heat up to high and bring to the boil with the lid on. Once it boils, reduce to a simmer and leave to cook for 25 minutes, stirring regularly to ensure the lentils don't stick to the bottom of the pot.

Check the seasoning and add more salt, pepper or lime juice if necessary. Roughly chop the fresh herbs.

Remove from the heat and add the spinach and the herbs before you serve. Garnish each bowl with a generous sprinkling of pickled ginger.

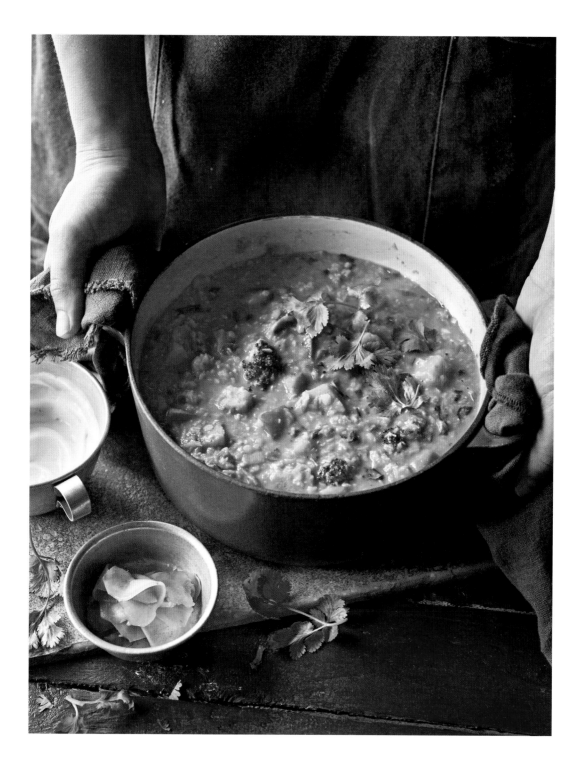

Tuscan Vegan Sausage and Bean Stew ♡ 🖐 ◌

This simple hearty one-pot dish is ideal to warm anyone up from the inside out. The bite of the vegan sausage goes really well with the soupy tomato-and-leek-based stew. This works great for batch cooking, as it freezes really well.

Serves 4–5
Takes 30 minutes

2 medium onions (250g)
3 cloves of garlic
1 fresh red chilli
25g fresh flat-leaf parsley
1 medium carrot (200g)
1 leek (300g)
2 x 400g tins of butter beans
    (approx. 480g when both
    drained)
300g vegan sausages
½ teaspoon dried thyme
1½ tablespoons tamari/
    soy sauce (make sure to
    use gf soy sauce if you
    need to avoid gluten)
1 teaspoon salt
400ml veg stock
1 x 400g tin of chopped
    tomatoes
2 teaspoons maple syrup
2 bay leaves
½ teaspoon ground
    black pepper
juice and zest of ½ a lime

Peel and finely chop the onions, garlic and chilli, and roughly chop the parsley. Cut the carrot and leek into small bite-size pieces. Drain and rinse the beans. Cut the vegan sausages into bite-size pieces.

Heat a non-stick pan over a high heat, and fry the sausages until they get a slight char on each side and are cooked through. If they start to stick, add a teaspoon of water and stir to loosen. Remove the cooked sausages from the pan and set aside.

Add the chopped onion, garlic and chilli to the pan and fry on a high heat for 4–5 minutes, until the onions start to brown and smell delicious (again, if they start to stick, add a teaspoon of water and stir to loosen).

Add the carrot and leek to the pan, with the thyme, tamari/soy sauce, a generous pinch of salt and about 50ml of the veg stock. Put a lid on the pan and cook for approximately 10–15 minutes, stirring occasionally to prevent the veg sticking and burning, until they are soft and nearly cooked through.

Add the butter beans, chopped tomatoes, the rest of the veg stock and salt, the maple syrup, bay leaves and black pepper. Bring to the boil, then reduce to a simmer and cook for approximately 5 minutes, or longer for a thicker sauce.

Taste the dish for seasoning before serving, and add salt, pepper, lime juice or chilli if required.

Serve sprinkled with the chopped parsley and with the vegan sausages on top – and enjoy!

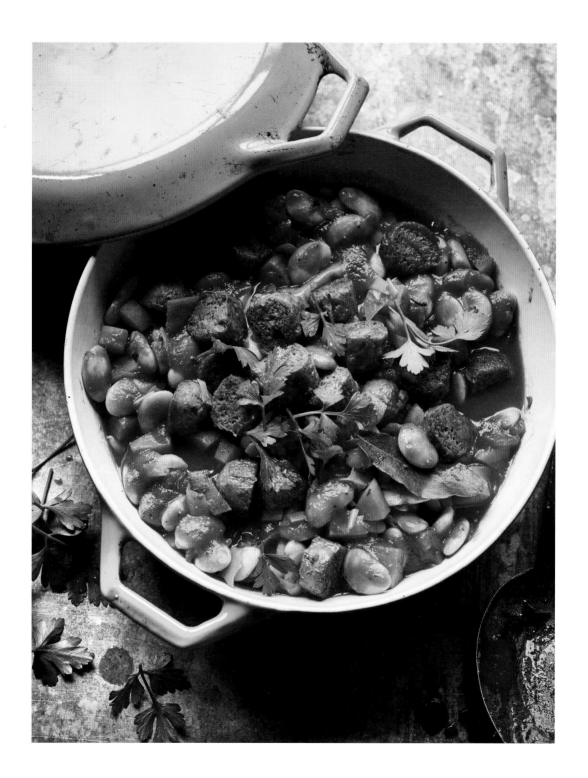

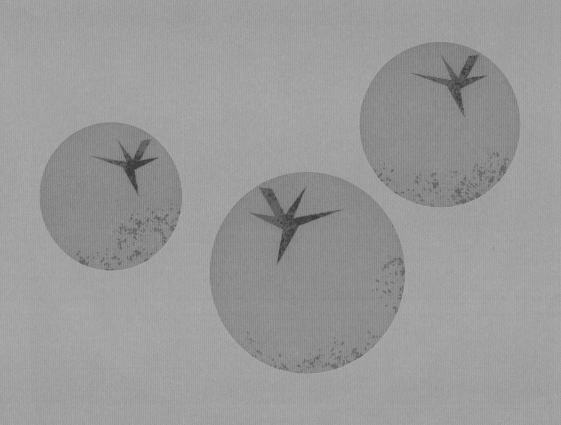

Chapter 14

Pasta Dinners

These are all crowd-pleasers and will satisfy the comfort eater within you! They're great family dishes that are healthier takes on their classic counterparts.

Easy Creamy Roasted Red Pepper Pasta ♡ ⓥ ⊘

So easy and tasty – the roasted red peppers add a lovely sweetness and a slight charred note that goes so well with the wholemeal pasta. This is pure creamy pasta deliciousness! Add any cooked veg you like to bulk this out, for example cooked broccoli, grilled courgettes, roasted cauliflower or fine beans.

Serves 4

Takes 15 minutes (plus soaking time)

300g wholemeal pasta of choice (use gluten-free if coeliac)

Red pepper sauce
100g cashew nuts
500ml oat milk
1½ teaspoons salt
¼ teaspoon ground black pepper
1 teaspoon garlic powder
juice of ½ a lemon
100g roasted red peppers (from a jar)

Veg
100g frozen peas
200g mushrooms
75g roasted red peppers (from a jar)
1 tablespoon tamari/ soy sauce (make sure to use gf soy sauce if you need to avoid gluten)
20g fresh basil

Drain and rinse the cashew nuts.

Put the frozen peas into a large bowl, cover with boiling water and leave to defrost. Finely chop the mushrooms. Slice the 75g of roasted red pepper into thin strips.

Soak the cashew nuts in boiling water for 10 minutes. Cook your pasta in well-salted water according to the packet instructions. While it is cooking, blend all the ingredients for the creamy red pepper sauce until nice and smooth.

Heat a non-stick pan on a high heat. Once hot, add the chopped mushrooms and fry for 5 minutes, stirring regularly. Once they start to brown, add the tamari/soy sauce and quickly stir it around the pan. Remove from the heat. Pick the basil leaves from their stalks.

Drain the pasta, keeping some of the cooking water aside. Drain and rinse the peas (make sure they are thawed). Add the drained pasta, peas, roasted red peppers (from a jar without the brine) and red pepper sauce to the cooked mushrooms, mix well over a medium heat until warmed through, adding a few tablespoons of pasta water to thin the sauce if needed, and simmer until the sauce has thickened nicely to your desired consistency.

Taste and season, then serve sprinkled with the basil leaves.

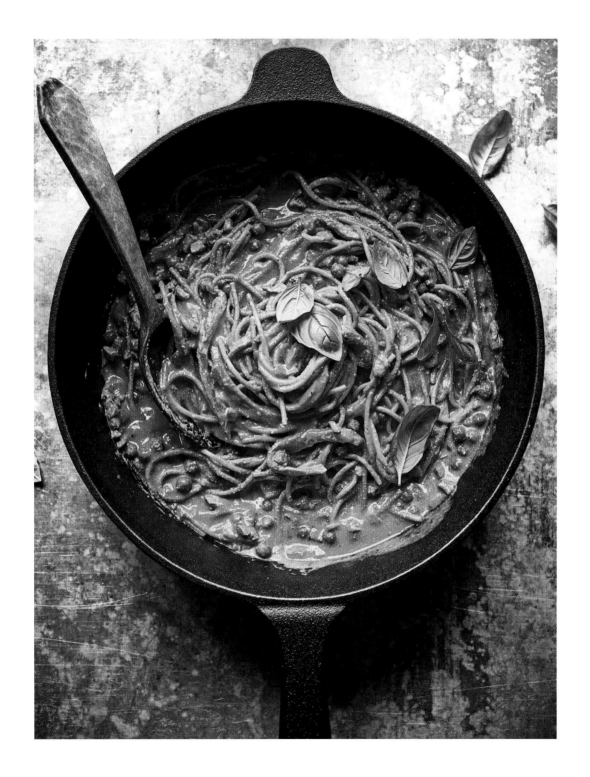

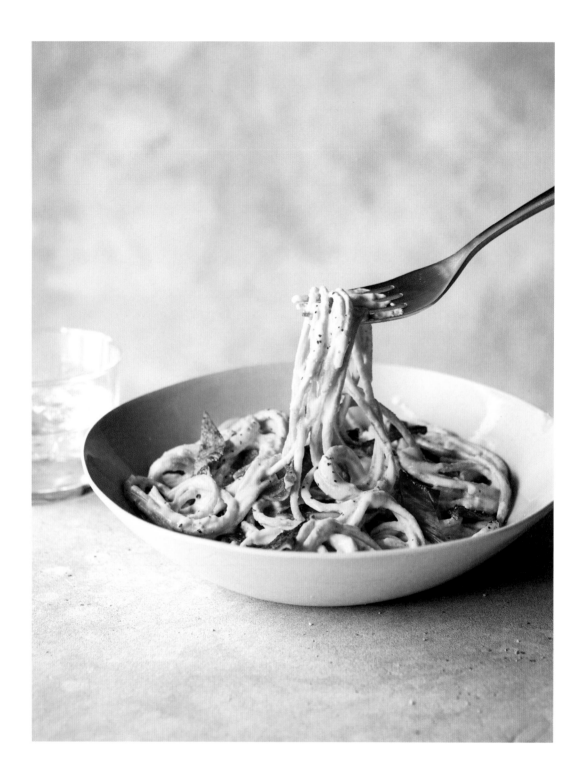

No Oil Creamy Carbonara ⊘ ⃠

Creamy, delicious, and the king oyster mushroom 'facon' is so good –
this is a fabulous dinner, no oil and lower-fat, but not lacking in flavour.
It makes a wonderful weekly dinner for any pasta lover.

Serves 3
Takes 15 minutes

300g wholemeal pasta (we
    use linguine or spaghetti
    – use wholemeal, or brown
    rice pasta for gluten-free)

Creamy sauce
50g cashew nuts
250ml oat milk
juice of ¼ of a lemon
½ teaspoon garlic powder
½ teaspoon salt

'Facon'
4 tablespoons tamari/
    soy sauce (make sure to
    use gf soy sauce if you
    need to avoid gluten)
2 tablespoons apple
    cider vinegar
2 tablespoons water
2 teaspoons maple syrup
2 teaspoons smoked paprika
3 tablespoons tomato purée
1 teaspoon garlic powder
a pinch of salt
2 king oyster mushrooms, or
    mushrooms of choice

Soak the cashew nuts in boiling water for 10 minutes, then drain and rinse. Put into a blender with the rest of the sauce ingredients and blend until lovely and smooth.

Cook the pasta in salted water according to the packet instructions and drain, keeping some of the cooking water (ideally pasta is cooked in water with the same salt content as sea water, which is 35g per litre – don't worry, most of this goes down the drain!).

In a bowl, mix together all the ingredients for the 'facon' apart from the king oyster mushrooms. Slice the mushrooms lengthwise into thin strips. Heat a non-stick pan on a high heat and add the sliced mushrooms. Using another similar-sized pan but slightly smaller, compress the mushrooms in the first pan for 2–3 minutes, until they start to brown. Turn over and repeat until they have browned on both sides.

Remove the mushrooms from the pan and add to the bowl of 'facon' marinade. Mix well. Reduce the heat of the pan to medium, put the marinated mushrooms back into the pan, and cook for about 1 minute on each side. Remove and set aside. Once cool, slice the mushrooms into thin strips about 1½cm wide.

Heat a clean non-stick pan on a high heat. Add a little of the sauce and the cooked pasta, then while stirring add the rest of the sauce and bring to the boil. Once hot, season to taste – if it starts to become too thick, add some of the reserved pasta water to reach the desired texture.

Garnish with lots of mushroom 'facon' and enjoy!

Spaghetti Bolognese ♡ ✋ ◌ ⊜

This is a lovely take on the traditional Italian pasta dish. It's quick to make and tastes amazing too. Nutritional yeast is a condiment that is available in all good health food stores. It brings a 'cheesy' taste to this dish, without any of the saturated fat. It's worth having in your cupboard. The wine adds a lovely depth of flavour here, and don't worry – the alcohol will burn off during the cooking process.

Serves 5
Takes 10–15 minutes

400g gluten-free spaghetti (brown rice is our favourite)
1 leek, green part only (approx. 200g)
1 large carrot (300g max)
1 fresh red chilli (leave out or reduce if you don't like spice)
400g tomatoes
200g cherry tomatoes
160g tinned cooked lentils
300g oyster mushrooms
2 teaspoons salt
2 tablespoons tamari/ soy sauce (make sure to use gf soy sauce if you need to avoid gluten)
2 tablespoons maple syrup
180ml red wine
1 x 400g tin of chopped tomatoes
salt and ground black pepper

To serve
a decent bunch of fresh basil
nutritional yeast

Cook the spaghetti according to the packet instructions, then drain and rinse under cold water to stop the pasta sticking together.

Finely chop the greens from the leek. Grate the carrot, and finely slice the chilli into small pieces. Finely chop the tomatoes and cut the cherry tomatoes in half. Drain and rinse the lentils. Finely chop the oyster mushrooms.

Heat a large non-stick pan on a high heat. Once the pan heats up, add the leek, chilli, grated carrot and 1 teaspoon of the salt. Cook for 3 minutes, stirring regularly. If it starts to stick, add a teaspoon of water and stir to loosen. Add the oyster mushrooms and cook for 3 minutes, stirring regularly. Add the tamari/soy sauce and cook for a further minute.

Next, add all the fresh tomatoes and the other teaspoon of salt, stir well, then add the lentils, maple syrup and red wine and cook for a further 3–4 minutes. Add the tinned tomatoes and bring to the boil, then reduce to a simmer and add the drained and rinsed pasta. Stir well, mixing everything thoroughly.

Pick the basil leaves from their stalks and set aside, then chop the basil stalks finely and add them to the pan.

Garnish with the basil leaves and scatter over some nutritional yeast.

Creamy Broccoli and Mushroom Pasta Bake ⊜

A really nourishing and super-delicious dinner which never lasts long in our households! The baked pasta goes crispy round the edges, which goes so well with the creamy white sauce.

Serves 6
Takes 25 minutes

200g dried gluten-free brown rice penne
1 bunch of spring onions/scallions, green parts only (50g)
1 large leek, green part only (150g)
200g oyster mushrooms
250g broccoli
2 tablespoons tamari/soy sauce (make sure to use gf soy sauce if you need to avoid gluten)
4 tablespoons water

Creamy sauce
5 tablespoons olive oil
5 tablespoons gluten-free flour
900ml almond milk
1 teaspoon salt
½ teaspoon ground black pepper
4 tablespoons nutritional yeast
a pinch of grated nutmeg
1 bay leaf

Topping
40g gluten-free breadcrumbs
1 tablespoon flaked almonds
a pinch of salt and ground black pepper
1 tablespoon olive oil

Preheat the oven to 200°C fan/220°C.

Cook the pasta according to the packet instructions.

While the pasta is cooking, chop the spring onion/scallion and leek greens (with the leeks, make sure to really clean them thoroughly, as sediment often hides inside). The white parts of the spring onions/scallions and leeks freeze well, and can be used for another dish. Finely chop the mushrooms and cut the broccoli into small bite-size florets.

Make the creamy sauce and cook the veg. Put the olive oil into a non-stick pan on a medium to high heat. When it's hot, sift in the flour and whisk for 2 minutes continuously until golden. Add the almond milk slowly, whisking until it all comes together. Add the rest of the sauce ingredients, bring to the boil, then reduce to a simmer. Being careful that nothing sticks to the bottom, simmer and whisk for 3–5 minutes. Once you have a smooth, creamy white sauce, remove the bay leaf, take the pan off the heat, then taste and add more salt if needed. Once the pasta is cooked, drain and rinse under cold water to stop the pasta sticking together.

Heat a large non-stick pan over a high heat. Once hot, add the green parts of the spring onions/scallions and leek, along with a good pinch of salt, and cook for 3 minutes, until the veg are softened. Add the mushrooms and tamari/soy sauce and cook for 5 minutes, until the mushrooms have reduced in volume and the tamari/soy sauce has been absorbed. If the veg starts to stick, add a teaspoon of water and stir to loosen. Add the broccoli and the water, reduce the heat to medium, cover tightly with a lid and steam until the broccoli is just cooked, about 5 minutes. Taste and make sure the broccoli is soft and cooked through.

Put the pasta, creamy sauce and cooked veg mixture into a large ovenproof baking dish about 32cm x 22cm. Mix together, then level out the surface. In a separate bowl mix all the topping ingredients together and scatter over the pasta bake. Pop into the preheated oven for 15 minutes, or until the top is golden brown.

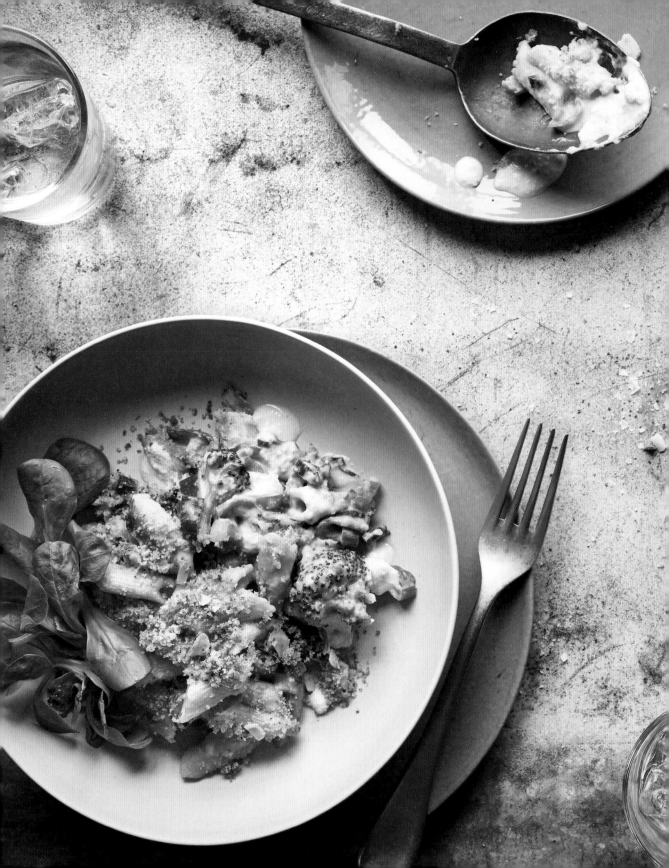

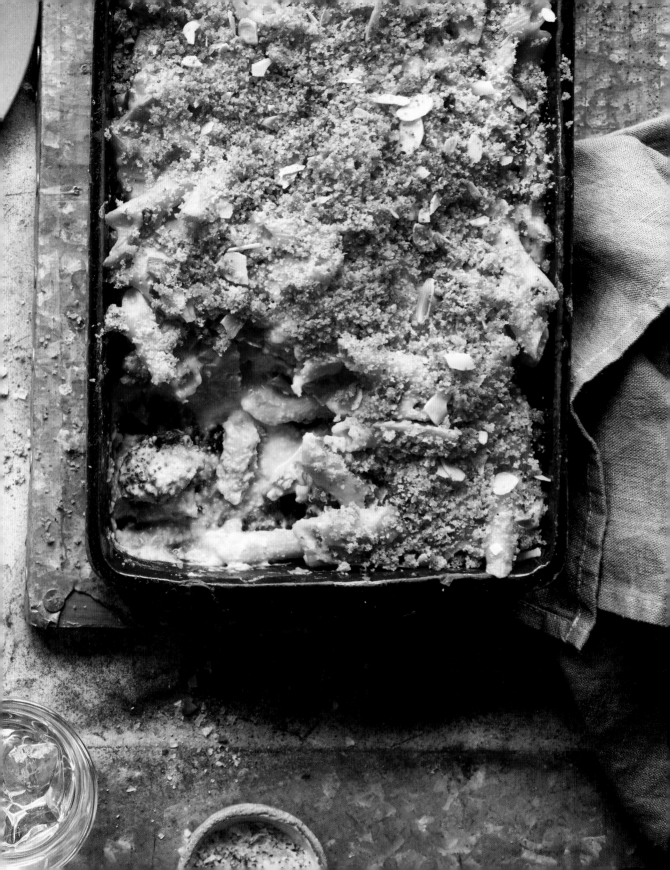

No Oil Creamy Lasagna ♡ ✋ ⊘

Traditionally a decadent treat of a dish – this recipe is based around whole plant foods and is every bit as good as its higher-fat version. This is really tasty and pretty straightforward to make.

Serves 6
Takes 55 minutes

500g dried lasagna sheets
    (you will need approx. 15
    – use wholewheat lasagna
    if you can)
fresh basil/flat-leaf parsley,
    to garnish

Tomato sauce
3 cloves of garlic
1 fresh red chilli
200g mushrooms of choice
400g sweet potatoes
100ml red wine
1 teaspoon salt
a few sprigs of fresh thyme
2 x 400g tins of chopped
    tomatoes
100g tomato purée
5 sun-dried tomatoes
1 bay leaf
1½ tablespoons maple syrup
ground black pepper

Béchamel
100g cashew nuts
400ml oat milk
juice of ½ a lemon
1 teaspoon garlic powder
1 teaspoon salt

Preheat the oven to 160°C fan/180°C.

Soak 5 lasagna sheets for the top layer so that they will cook properly. To do so, lay out your 5 wholemeal lasagna sheets in a baking or roasting tin, pour over boiling water and leave to soak. Ensure the sheets are well spread out so that they won't stick together.

Peel and finely chop the garlic and chilli (include the seeds if you like it spicier). Cut the mushrooms and sweet potatoes into bite-size pieces, keeping the skin on. Put the cashew nuts into a bowl, cover with boiling water, and leave to soak for 10 minutes.

Heat a large, wide-bottomed non-stick pan on a high heat. Once hot, add the chilli and garlic and fry for 1 minute, stirring continuously. Add the chopped mushrooms and sweet potatoes, the red wine and a generous pinch of salt, and mix well. Put a lid on the pan and leave to cook for 12–15 minutes, stirring occasionally. Once the sweet potatoes are soft, remove the thyme leaves from their stalks and add to the pan with the rest of the sauce ingredients. Mix well, bring to the boil, then reduce to a simmer for 5 minutes. Taste and adjust the seasoning with salt and ground black pepper. Take off the heat and set aside.

To make the béchamel, drain and rinse the cashew nuts. Put them into a blender with the rest of the béchamel ingredients and blend until nice and smooth.

To assemble the lasagna, put a thin layer of béchamel on the bottom of a large ovenproof baking dish about 32cm x 22cm, spreading it out evenly. Add a single even layer of dried lasagna sheets. Next add a layer of your tomato sauce, then another layer of lasagna sheets. Repeat with one more layer of tomato sauce, then a final layer of lasagna sheets (using the soaked lasagna sheets last). Spread the remaining béchamel sauce on top, making sure the lasagna sheets are completely covered.

Bake in the preheated oven for 20–25 minutes, until the lasagna sheets are cooked and the dish is bubbling.

Remove the lasagna from the oven and sprinkle over the herbs.

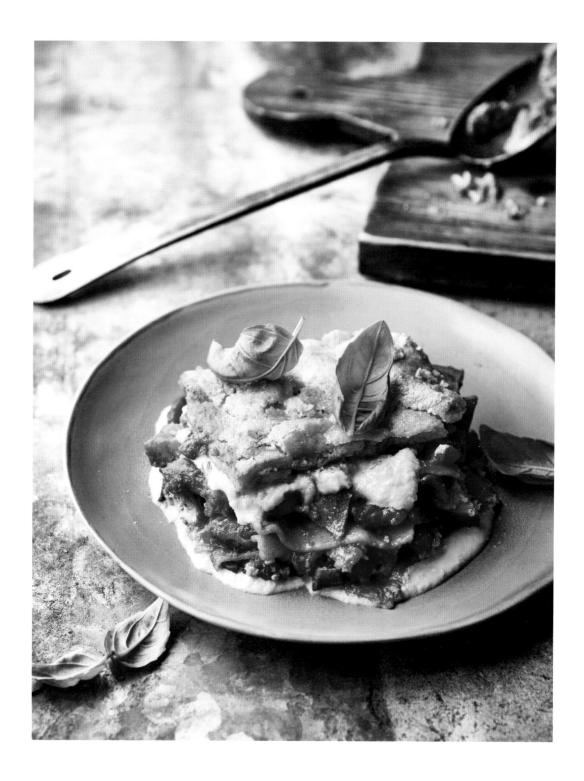

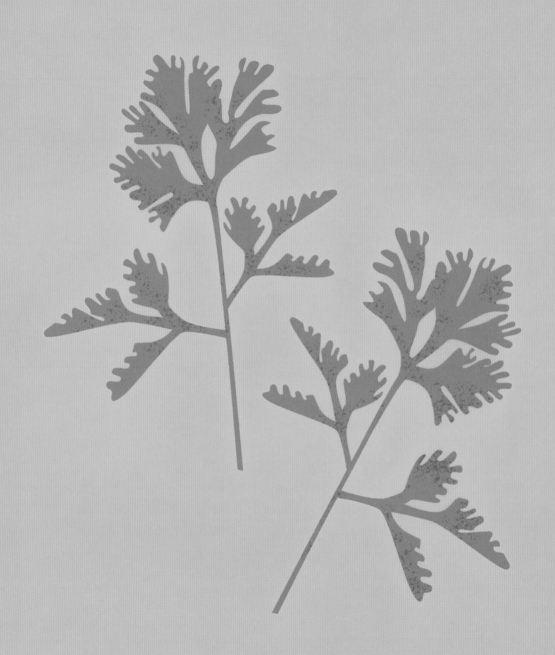

Chapter 15

Centrepiece Meals

These dishes work great whatever the occasion – they will leave your guests looking for more, and more importantly, you will feel light and happy that you stayed on track.

Cottage Pie with Sweet Potato Mash and Coriander Drizzle ♡ 🖐 ⃠

This simple bake tastes even better on day two! Serve with a simple green salad. It tastes like a belly hug and makes a wonderful family dinner or a cold lunch the next day.

Serves 6–8
Takes 60 minutes

2 medium carrots or parsnips
100g green beans
3 x 400g tins of cooked Puy lentils, or other green or brown lentils
6 sprigs of fresh thyme
2 bay leaves
a pinch of salt
3 tablespoons tamari/ soy sauce (make sure to use gf soy sauce if you need to avoid gluten)
750ml veg stock
½ teaspoon ground black pepper

Mash
750g sweet potatoes
250g potatoes
1 teaspoon salt
100ml non-dairy milk
a pinch of ground black pepper

Coriander cream
100g cashew nuts
65ml water
15g fresh coriander
⅓ teaspoon garlic powder
½ teaspoon salt
1 teaspoon balsamic vinegar

Preheat the oven to 180°C fan/200°C.

Put the cashew nuts into a bowl, cover with boiling water and leave to soak for 10 minutes.

Chop the sweet potatoes and regular potatoes into uniform bite-size pieces so that they will cook evenly. Put them into a medium pan, cover with water, bring to the boil and cook until soft, about 20–25 minutes.

Grate the carrots or parsnips. Trim the green beans and cut them in half. Drain and rinse the lentils. Pick the leaves off the thyme sprigs.

Put another medium pan on a high heat and add the grated carrot or parsnip. Add the thyme leaves, bay leaves and a pinch of salt, mix well, and cook for 3 minutes, stirring occasionally. Add the drained lentils and the tamari/soy sauce, then slowly add the veg stock. Add the black pepper, bring to the boil, then reduce to a simmer, letting the stock slowly evaporate for 10 minutes, stirring occasionally.

Meanwhile, make the coriander cream. Drain and rinse the soaked cashew nuts. Put them into a blender with the rest of the coriander cream ingredients (reserving a few coriander leaves for garnish) and blend until nice and smooth.

If the lentil mixture is dry once it has thickened, add 2 tablespoons of water and ½ tablespoon of tamari/soy sauce and season. Add the green beans and stir them through the hot lentil mixture, letting them cook for a minute or two. Remove from the heat and set aside.

Drain the potatoes, then put them back into the pan and add 1 teaspoon of salt, pepper and milk. Mash it all together until lovely and smooth.

Remove the bay leaves from the lentil and veg mixture, then spoon into a 28cm x 20cm baking dish. Drizzle over half the coriander cream, and distribute the sweet potato mash evenly on top. Bake in the preheated oven for 25 minutes, until the top crisps.

Before serving, drizzle over the rest of the coriander cream and garnish with the reserved coriander leaves.

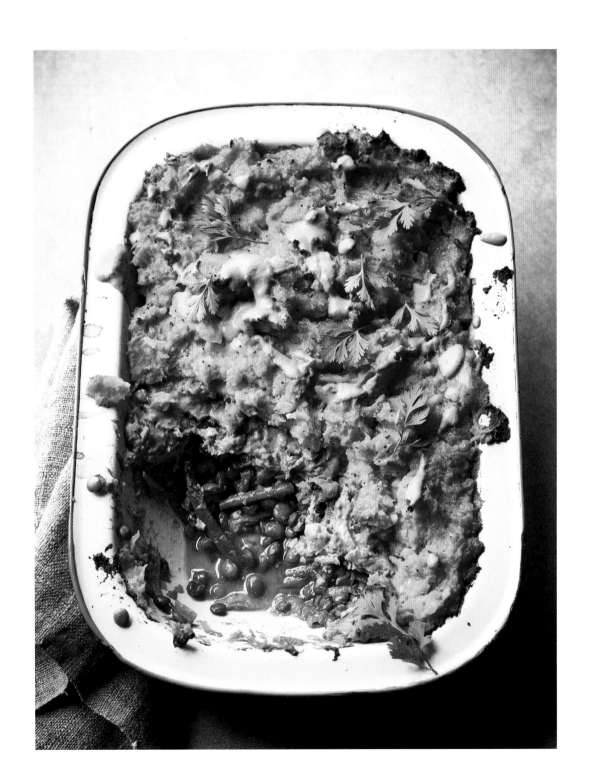

Greek Spanakopita with Sweet Potato ♡ 🤚 ⃠

This dish is well worth the effort – it makes a lovely cold lunch or a piping hot winter centrepiece meal. Although this is a lower-fat version it's still 4% above the recommended 10% fat content – but well worth it as an occasional treat.

Serves 4–6
Takes 50 minutes

2 sheets of vegan puff
   pastry (640g)
1 leek (both the white
   and green parts)
   (approx. 200g)
400g frozen spinach
400g sweet potatoes
15g fresh dill
15g fresh mint
1 teaspoon salt
100ml veg stock
a pinch of grated nutmeg
½ teaspoon ground
   black pepper
zest and juice of ½ a lemon
non-dairy milk, for brushing

Quick-fire cashew feta
150g cashew nuts
2 tablespoons lemon juice
¾ teaspoon salt
1 tablespoon non-dairy milk

Defrost the puff pastry if frozen. Preheat the oven to 200°C fan/220°C.

Fill and boil the kettle. Put the cashew nuts into a bowl, cover with boiling water, and leave to soak for 10 minutes. Chop the leek lengthwise and wash the inside thoroughly, as sediment often hides in the green part of the leek. Finely slice the leek. Put the spinach into a bowl and defrost it by pouring boiling water over it and leaving it to sit for a few minutes. Cut the sweet potato into bite-size pieces, keeping the skin on and removing any blemishes. Finely chop the dill and mint leaves.

Heat a wide-bottomed non-stick pan on a high heat. Once hot, add the chopped leek and cook for 4 minutes, until it starts to brown slightly, stirring regularly. If it starts to stick, add a teaspoon of water and stir to loosen. Drain the spinach and add to the pan along with the chopped sweet potatoes, salt and 100ml of veg stock. Mix well, then put a lid on the pan and leave to steam for 10–15 minutes, until the sweet potatoes are soft.

Add the dill and mint, nutmeg, ground black pepper and lemon juice and zest to the sweet potatoes, and mix well. Take the pan off the heat.

Drain and rinse the cashew nuts. Put them into a blender along with the rest of the cashew feta ingredients and pulse until it starts to crumble but does not become a sauce. This should take only 30–40 seconds. Add the cashew feta to the spinach and sweet potato mixture and carefully fold it in. Taste and adjust the seasoning with more salt, pepper or lemon juice.

Line a baking tray about 32cm x 22cm x 6cm with parchment paper. Lay a sheet of pastry in the tray, to cover the base, ensuring that it comes up the sides. Add the spinach and cashew feta mixture and gently compact, spreading it out evenly. Top with the second layer of pastry, making sure that the edges are sealed and there is a single layer of pastry covering the filling.

Using a pastry brush, gently brush the outside of the pastry with a light coating of oat milk. Bake in the preheated oven for 20–25 minutes, until the pastry is golden.

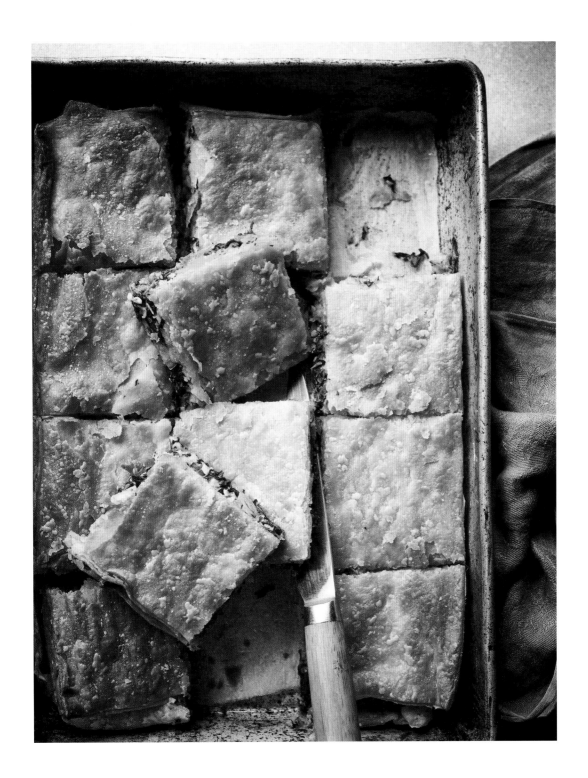

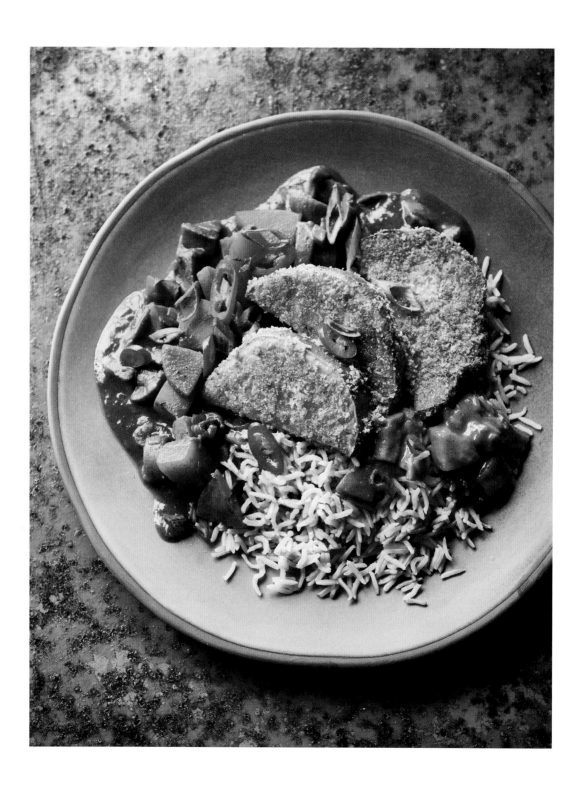

Katsu Curry ♡ ✋ ⊘

Here we make a breaded crispy sweet potato cutlet in place of the traditional breaded pork, which adds a lovely crispy sweet bite to elevate the curry. This makes a dinner well worth the effort!

Serves 4–5
Takes 50 minutes

1 teaspoon oil
350g uncooked brown basmati or short-grain brown rice

Breaded sweet potato cutlets (makes about 12)
1 large sweet potato (approx. 600g)
a pinch of salt
1 tablespoon ground flax seeds
100g plain white flour
100ml non-dairy milk
80g brown breadcrumbs

Curry
200g mushrooms
2 carrots (200g)
2 stalks of celery
1 medium onion
400g potatoes
½ a thumb-size piece of fresh ginger
2 cloves of garlic
3 tablespoons curry powder
2 tablespoons garam masala
½ teaspoon ground cinnamon
675ml veg stock
2 tablespoons coconut sugar or brown sugar
1 teaspoon salt
1 tablespoon tamari/soy sauce (use gf if you avoid gluten)
1 tablespoon vinegar

Garnish
spring onions/scallions (green parts only)
fresh red chillies

Preheat the oven to 180°C fan/200°C.

Cut the sweet potato lengthwise into thin wedges and put them on a baking tray. Add a generous pinch of salt and roast in the preheated oven for 20 minutes, or until nearly cooked through.

Peel the onion and then chop it into bite-size pieces along with the mushrooms, carrots, celery and potatoes. Slice the spring onions/scallions and chillies. Cook the rice according to the packet directions. Peel and finely chop the ginger and garlic.

Put a large non-stick pan on a high heat. Once hot, add the carrots, celery, onion, ginger and garlic and cook for 5–8 minutes, stirring regularly, until the carrots are starting to cook through. If they start to stick, add a teaspoon of water and stir to loosen. Add the mushrooms, mix well, then add the spices, stirring well for 1 minute to release the flavour.

Add the stock, sugar, salt, tamari/soy sauce, vinegar and chopped potatoes, bring to a simmer, then cover with a tight lid and cook for 15–20 minutes, until the potatoes are soft and the sauce has thickened. Reduce to a gentle simmer before serving.

For the sweet potato cutlets, make your flax egg according to the instructions on page 102. Set up your breading station: put the flour, the flax egg and milk, and the breadcrumbs on three separate large plates. Dip the sweet potato first into the flour, then into the flax egg/milk, then into the breadcrumbs, until well coated. Repeat until you have coated all the sweet potato pieces.

Heat a non-stick frying pan on a high heat. Once hot, add 1 teaspoon of oil and wipe it round the pan using a piece of kitchen paper to remove most of the oil. Reduce the heat to medium and add the breaded sweet potato pieces a few at a time so that each one has enough space to fry properly. Turn so that they brown on all sides. Repeat until all are cooked. Remove the sweet potato from the pan and set aside on kitchen paper.

Serve your finished katsu curry with rice and some of the sweet potato cutlets, sprinkled with spring onions/scallions and chillies.

Centrepiece Meals

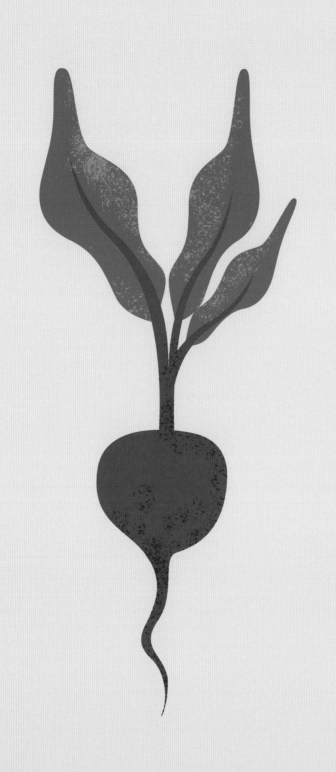

Chapter 16

Snacks

We are serious snackers, so we have
you covered in this section. These are all low
in calories and high in fibre.

Kale Crisps ♡ ✋ ⊘ 😊

Kale crisps are a super-nutritious and tasty snack – they are next level potato chips! The recipe below is for spicy kale chips, but if you prefer, simply leave out the spices and add a generous pinch of sea salt instead. It's a wonderful way to get more greens!

Serves 2
Takes 25 minutes

200g kale (approx. 100g weight without stalks)
2 tablespoons tamari/ soy sauce (make sure to use gf soy sauce if you need to avoid gluten)
1 tablespoon lemon juice
½ teaspoon paprika
a pinch of cayenne pepper, or more (e.g. ½ teaspoon) if you like it spicy
a light sprinkling of salt
2 tablespoons nutritional yeast

Preheat the oven to 100°C fan/120°C.

Remove the kale leaves from the thick central stalks. Give them a thorough wash and dry.

Mix the tamari/soy sauce and lemon juice and massage it right through the kale, making sure you coat each leaf. Add the spices, a pinch of salt and the nutritional yeast and mix well.

Lay the leaves on a baking tray, making sure they are well spread out so that they will crisp up, and bake in the preheated oven for 15–20 minutes, until nice and crispy. Halfway through the cooking time, give the kale a good mix around to ensure your chips are all crisping up evenly.

Leave to cool for 3 minutes on the tray. These are best eaten when they are fresh out of the oven, but they can be stored in an airtight container for 2–3 days.

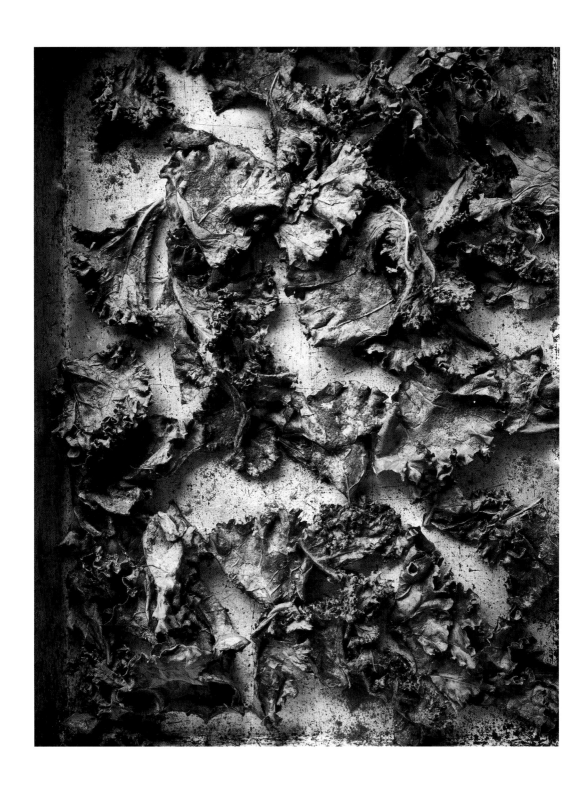

Happy Gut Hummus ♡ ✋ ⊘ ⊜

This is a really tasty basic low-FODMAP hummus. It doesn't have any garlic in it, as garlic is high in fructans and is therefore a high-FODMAP food. This goes great on top of toasted gluten-free pittas, rice cakes, or our gluten-free porridge bread (see page 134). Make sure to adjust the seasoning as you see fit by adding more lemon, cumin, chilli, etc. until it becomes the perfect hummus for you! This recipe makes 9 portions – each portion is 2 tablespoons or 40g.

Makes 375g
Takes 10 minutes

1 x 400g tin of
   chickpeas
   (approx. 240g
   when drained)
juice of 1 lemon
   (40ml)
45g light tahini
1 teaspoon salt

a pinch of ground
   black pepper
½ teaspoon ground
   cumin
a pinch of chilli flakes
   (optional – if you
   like it hot)
9 tablespoons water

Drain the chickpeas and rinse thoroughly, then put them into a food processor together with the rest of the ingredients and blend for about 3 minutes, until pretty smooth.

In spite of it not having any garlic, this is a really tasty recipe. Taste and season with more salt and pepper if you think it needs it, and as there is no garlic maybe try the chilli flakes if you like a little spice.

Lower-in-fat Hummus
3 ways ♡ ✋ ⊘

This is a really tasty lower-in-fat hummus. It contains no refined foods and is a lighter, full-flavoured hummus. It's a nice basic recipe, and opposite we include two variations to give you an idea of the directions you could take your hummus creations!

Makes 400g
Takes 10 minutes

1 x 400g tin of
   chickpeas
   (approx. 240g
   when drained)
juice of 1 lemon
   (40ml)
65g light tahini

1 teaspoon salt
a pinch of ground
   black pepper
½ teaspoon ground
   cumin
12 tablespoons water
a pinch of chilli flakes
   (optional, if you
   like it hot)

Drain the chickpeas and rinse thoroughly, then put them into a food processor together with the rest of the ingredients and blend for about 3 minutes, until pretty smooth.

Taste and season with more salt and pepper if you think it needs it.

Roasted Red Pepper Smoked Hummus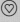

Makes 375g
Takes 10 minutes

1 x 400g tin of
  chickpeas
  (approx. 240g
  when drained)
100g roasted red
  peppers (in brine,
  from a jar)
juice of 1 lemon
  (40ml)
65g light tahini

1 teaspoon salt
a pinch of ground
  black pepper
½ teaspoon ground
  cumin
a pinch of chilli flakes
  (optional, if you
  like it hot)
4 tablespoons water
⅓ teaspoon smoked
  paprika
1 teaspoon maple
  syrup

Drain the chickpeas and rinse thoroughly, and drain the
red peppers of their brine, then put them into a food
processor together with the rest of the ingredients and
blend for about 3 minutes, until pretty smooth.

Taste and season with more salt and pepper if you think
it needs it.

Sweet Beet Hummus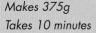

Makes 375g
Takes 10 minutes

1 x 400g tin of
  chickpeas
  (approx. 240g
  when drained)
zest of 1 lemon
juice of 1 lemon
  (40ml)

65g light tahini
1 teaspoon salt
a pinch of ground
  black pepper
100g cooked
  beetroot
  (vac-packed)
4 tablespoons water
½ teaspoon maple
  syrup

Drain the chickpeas and rinse thoroughly, then put
them into a food processor together with the rest of
the ingredients and blend for about 3 minutes, until
pretty smooth.

Taste and season with more salt and pepper if you
think it needs it.

Buckwheat Flatbread

Here is a simple gluten-free buckwheat flatbread, with some suggestions for adding more character. We use buckwheat because, in spite of its name, it does not contain any gluten. It's actually a seed and is also known as a pseudo-grain.

Makes 6 small flatbreads
Takes 20 minutes

140ml cold water
240g buckwheat flour
2 tablespoons baking powder
1 teaspoon salt

Pour the water into a large bowl, sieve in the flour, and add the baking powder and salt. Bring together into a dough – no need to knead it, just make sure it's well mixed.

Divide the dough into six pieces. Take one piece and shape into a flat disc. Carefully roll out the dough into a round flatbread shape about ½cm thick. Pierce the dough with a fork a few times, and dust lightly with buckwheat flour or gluten-free flour.

Heat a non-stick frying pan on a medium heat. Once it's hot, add one of the flatbreads and cook for 3–4 minutes, until it starts to brown slightly and create some bubbles. Carefully turn it around and do the same with the other side. Repeat with the rest of the flatbreads.

These work great with hummus, sauerkraut, cucumber and any other fillings of choice (making sure that they are also low-FODMAP).

Optional additions for 6 flatbreads (mix these into the dough before cooking):

- 5 tablespoons of sesame seeds and 3 tablespoons of mixed herbs for a Middle Eastern note.

- 1 tablespoon of sumac adds a nice citrus undertone.

- 1 teaspoon of chilli powder – to spice it up.

- ½ teaspoon of smoked paprika for a nice smoky undertone.

- 1 tablespoon of cumin seeds, with ½ teaspoon of fennel seeds for a musky aniseed flavour.

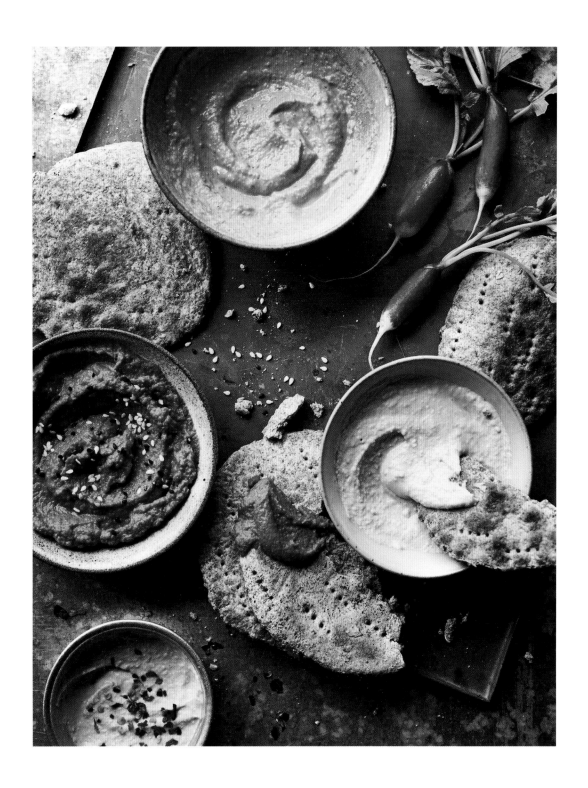

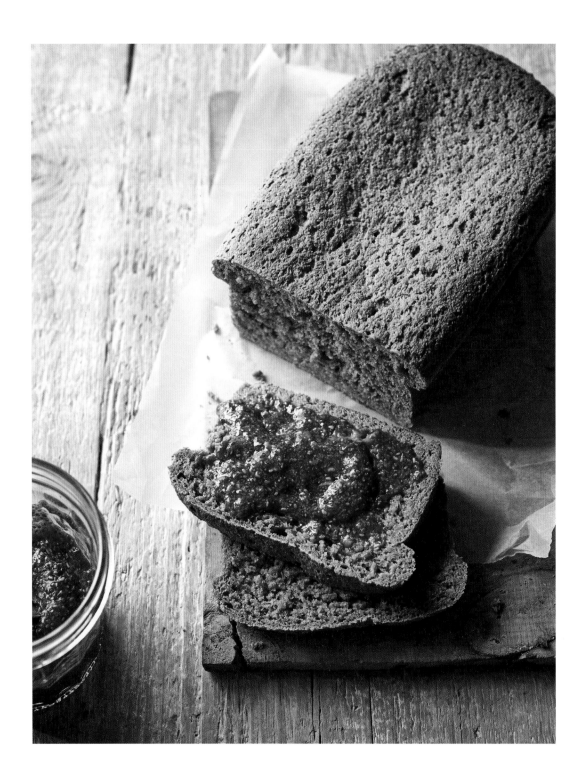

Malted Yeast Bread ♡ ✋ ⊘

The malted flour gives this bread a lovely sweet earthiness. This is a relatively simple bread to make, in that you just knead, leave to rise and then bake. Once the bread is cool, you can cut it in slices and freeze it in freezer bags, so that when you're stuck you can simply take it out of the freezer, toast it, and you have some fresh healthy bread!

Makes 1 x 500g loaf
Takes 60 minutes

325ml warm water
7g fast-action yeast
350g wholewheat flour
150g malt flour
12g salt

Put the water into a large bowl. Ideally, the water should be around body temperature. Add the yeast and mix it around, then pour in the two types of flour and the salt and mix until it comes together.

Pour the mixture out on the work surface (no need to flour it) and knead for 8–10 minutes, until you develop what is known as the windowpane effect. This means that when you stretch the dough and hold it up to the light, the light should shine through like a windowpane. If it rips it needs to be kneaded for longer until you reach this effect.

Line a 1lb loaf tin with baking parchment. Put in the dough and leave to rise for 3 hours, covered with a damp tea towel. It should almost double in volume.

Preheat the oven to 180°C fan/200°C. Bake the bread for 35 minutes, then take out, remove from the tin and leave to cool on a wire rack before slicing.

We like to eat this toasted, with chia jam (see page 135).

Chapter 17

Healthier Desserts

As the title suggests, these are indeed
healthier dishes to fit with our plans. They will scratch
that sweet itch you may have, so enjoy knowing
that these treats are doing you good!

Skinny Banana Bread ⊜

This banana bread is more like a fruit brack than a cake – it's light and sweet, and fairly simple to make. For best results, bake it in a shallow pie dish or brownie tray so that it cooks through fully, rather than a loaf tin. It's a lovely healthy snack that goes great with a cup of tea or coffee.

Makes 12 squares
Takes 60 minutes

3 large greenish bananas
  (preferably not ripe, as you
  want them to be low-
  FODMAP, see page 86)
90ml rice milk or almond milk
160ml maple syrup
2 tablespoons molasses
240g buckwheat flour or
  gluten-free flour
½ tablespoon baking powder
¾ teaspoon bicarbonate
  of soda
1 teaspoon ground cinnamon
¼ teaspoon grated nutmeg
½ teaspoon salt
50g raisins, soaked for
  5 minutes in water
  (optional, for a juicier bite)
20g pumpkin seeds

Preheat the oven to 150°C fan/170°C.

Mash the bananas really well. Put them into a food processor with the rest of the ingredients (apart from the raisins and pumpkin seeds), and blend until everything is well mixed (if you don't have a food processor, mix the wet ingredients and the dry ingredients separately and then combine them). Drain the raisins, then put them into a large bowl with the banana mixture and mix well.

Line a flat pie dish/brownie type tray (28cm x 18cm x 4cm) with baking parchment. Pour in the mixture and spread out evenly. Sprinkle with the pumpkin seeds and bake in the preheated oven for 50 minutes, until a knife inserted in the centre of the loaf comes out clean.

Remove from the oven and carefully take the banana bread out of the tin. Allow to cool on a wire rack before slicing.

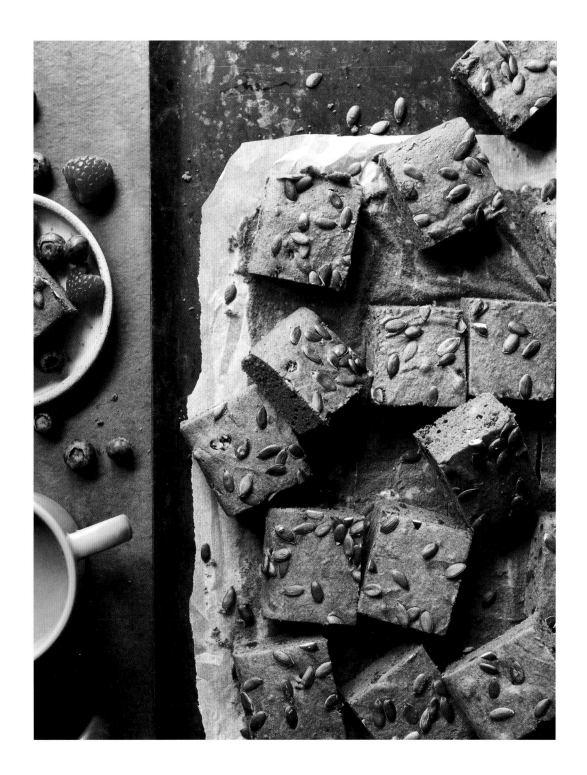

Energy Balls 2 Ways

Tropical Energy Balls ♡ ✋ ⊘

A few years back we made a quick variation of these with a yoga friend, Patrick Beach. We forgot to write down the recipe and never published the video, so here's an even better version. Toasting the coconut means it caramelizes slightly and adds more flavour, and we also soak the mango and goji berries to rehydrate them and make them easier to blend. These are delicious, and make a wonderful healthy snack.

Makes 18 x 20g balls
Takes 15 minutes

150g dried mango
60g goji berries
100ml orange juice or
    pineapple juice
70g desiccated coconut
30g pumpkin seeds
80g oat flakes (use gluten-free
    if coeliac)
30g peanut butter
1 teaspoon ground cinnamon
    (optional)
zest of 1 orange

Use scissors to cut the dried mango into small pieces. Put them into a bowl with the goji berries, then cover with the orange or pineapple juice and leave to sit for 5 minutes.

Heat a non-stick pan on a medium heat. Once warm, add 50g of desiccated coconut and toast until it starts to turn golden, stirring regularly. Once golden and smelling wonderful, remove from the pan and set aside.

Roughly chop the pumpkin seeds until they start to break up into smaller pieces. Put into a food processor with the rest of the ingredients apart from the remaining coconut, including the soaked dried mango and goji berries and the juice. Blend until they start to come together. If you want a smooth homogeneous energy ball, blend for longer – if you want a multicoloured textured ball, pulse just until it starts to come together. The mango can be very firm, so you may have to blend for a little longer, depending on your food processor.

Using a spoon and clean hands, roll the filling into smooth 20g balls. Roll them in the untoasted desiccated coconut. They will keep for 5–7 days in the fridge.

Chocolate Hazelnut Delights ♡ ✋ ⃠

This is a healthier take on Nutella-filled truffle pralines. It's worth seeking out some hazelnut butter or hazelnut milk, as these will give you the subtle yet distinctive flavour of hazelnut and chocolate. Medjool dates can seem a little pricey, but they are so worth it and really do make a difference to the texture of these balls. Enjoy – these are a delightful healthier treat!

Makes 20 x 20g balls
Takes 15 minutes

100g oat flakes
2 tablespoons cocoa powder
200g medjool dates
50ml hazelnut milk
60g hazelnut butter
1 teaspoon vanilla extract
a pinch of salt

To garnish
10g freeze-dried raspberries

Put the oat flakes and cocoa powder into a food processor or blender and blend until the oats start to become like flour. If your food processor or blender can't do this, don't worry!

Remove the stones from the dates. Add the dates to the food processor along with the rest of the ingredients apart from the raspberries and blend until wonderfully smooth.

Using a spoon and clean hands, roll the filling into smooth table-tennis size balls.

Crush the freeze-dried raspberries to a powder. Roll each ball in the raspberry powder. They will keep for 5–7 days in the fridge.

Healthier Hot Chocolate

Like a warm belly hug, this hot chocolate is perfect on a cold winter's evening or simply when you need it! The orange zest works great to elevate it and give it another dimension (but if you're a mint lover rather than an orange choc lover, it's worth seeking out some mint oil).

Serves 2 (makes about 400ml)

Takes 5 minutes

300ml rice milk or almond milk
2 tablespoons cocoa powder
1 teaspoon vanilla extract
2 tablespoons maple syrup
1 tablespoon smooth almond butter (use chunky if you prefer chunks!)
zest of ½ an orange or 1–2 drops of mint oil (optional) for a minty hot chocolate – you can even add a mint tea bag when heating up and remove it before serving
a tiny pinch of salt

Place a saucepan on a medium heat and add the milk, then slowly add the remainder of the ingredients as you heat the milk.

Continue to heat the chocolate liquid on a medium heat, stirring continuously with a whisk, until the mixture is smooth and creamy and at the temperature you would like.

We love this with the extra texture from the almond butter and orange zest, but if you prefer a smoother hot chocolate, pour it through a sieve to remove any little pieces before serving.

Maple and Seed Flapjack ☺

These flapjack bars make a tasty and healthy snack on the go, and they are packed with fibre and goodness too. Dave's daughters get them as a treat for school and love them! Sometimes if you don't compact these well enough or don't leave them to cool they can become crumbly – don't worry, you can enjoy them as granola instead.

Makes 12 flapjacks
Takes 50 minutes

250g gluten-free oats
160ml coconut oil
70g ground flax seeds
160ml maple syrup
40g desiccated coconut
40g pumpkin seeds
40g sunflower seeds
40g sesame seeds
40g ground almonds
40g raisins
a pinch of salt

Put the oats into a bowl and mix with the oil, so that the oats are well coated. Add all the remaining ingredients and mix well.

Line a standard flapjack tray (28cm x 18cm x 4cm) with baking parchment.

Roll out the mix on the baking tray, to around 2½cm thick. Make sure you compact it well, so that it stays together once baked.

Bake at 140°C fan/160°C for 35–40 minutes, until lightly golden. Leave to cool, then cut into 12 pieces.

Berry Crumble ☺

This crumble recipe is dairy-, gluten- and refined sugar-free, and it's super-tasty too. Be careful – if you try it, you might end up eating half of it in one go! If you are making this when rhubarb is in season, feel free to use rhubarb instead of strawberries, as in this quantity it's low-FODMAP too.

Serves 8
Takes 30 minutes

Stewed fruit
800g strawberries (if using frozen strawberries, let them thaw first), or 800g rhubarb
200g raspberries
4 tablespoons water
5 tablespoons maple syrup
2 teaspoons ground cinnamon
1 teaspoon ground ginger

Crumble
75ml sunflower oil/coconut oil (5 tablespoons)
150g gluten-free oats
50g ground almonds
3 tablespoons pumpkin seeds
3 tablespoons sunflower seeds
90ml maple syrup

If using rhubarb, cut it into bite-size pieces and put them into a pan with the berries. If just using berries, put them into a pan along with the 4 tablespoons of water, the maple syrup, ground cinnamon and ground ginger. Bring the fruit mixture to the boil, then reduce to a simmer with the lid on. Stirring occasionally, stew the fruit for about 20 minutes, or until it has all properly broken down.

In the meantime, preheat the oven to 170°C fan/190°C.

If using coconut oil for the crumble, melt it first by heating it in a pan. Thoroughly mix all the ingredients for the crumble together in a bowl, including the oil.

Once the fruit has broken down, put it into your crumble dish and spread it out evenly (we use a 30cm ceramic dish). Spread the crumble mixture evenly over the fruit and bake in the preheated oven for about 25 minutes, or until the top of the crumble starts to turn golden.

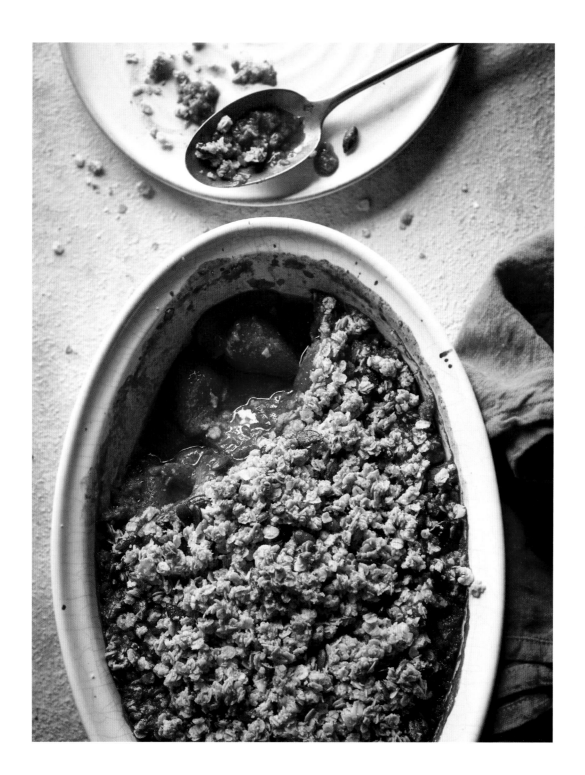

4 Simple Healthier Dessert Sauces

Here are four simple sauces which can transform a boring snack into something that feels more indulgent. They are all below 10% fat and are based around wholefoods, so they are definitely in the healthy snack category.

Each of these makes approx. 300g and takes 10–15 minutes.

Simple Date Caramel ♡ 🖐 ⊘

Simple and delicious – goes great on top of sliced fruit, spread on toast for a sweet spread, on top of your porridge or even just eaten straight up with a spoon!

150g pitted dates or
    medjool dates
100ml boiling water
½ teaspoon vanilla extract
2 tablespoons almond butter
a pinch of salt

If you have time, soak the dates in the boiling water for 5 minutes. Drain them, remove the stones, then put them into a food processor or blender with the rest of the ingredients and blend until smooth.

This goes great served on sliced apple with some coconut yoghurt! Keeps for up to 1 week in an airtight container in the fridge.

Chocolate Sauce ♡ 🖐 ⊘

We love this spread over hot toast, and it also makes a wonderful topping for porridge. The chocolate spread came from a man doing our Happy Heart course – he used to add more water to our energy balls recipe to make them runnier, then spread them on his toast – we thought this was ingenious, so this one is for him!

150g pitted dates or
    medjool dates
100ml boiling water
4 tablespoons cocoa powder
½ teaspoon vanilla extract
2 tablespoons almond butter
a pinch of salt

If you have time, soak the dates for 5 minutes in the boiling water. Drain them, then remove the stones. Put them into a food processor or blender with the rest of the ingredients and blend until smooth. If you want to make it even smoother and thicker, just put everything into a pan and heat on a gentle heat until it reaches your desired texture, while stirring continuously.

This will keep for up to 1 week in an airtight container in the fridge.

Hazelnut Chocolate Spread

This is a much healthier take on the ever-popular chocolate hazelnut spread – goes wonderful on fresh bread or toast, or even eaten straight off the spoon!

150g pitted dates or
    medjool dates
100ml boiling water
80ml hazelnut milk
2 tablespoons hazelnut butter
1 tablespoon cocoa powder
½ teaspoon vanilla extract
a pinch of salt

If you have time, soak the dates for 5 minutes in the boiling water. Drain them, remove the stones, then put them into a food processor or blender with the rest of the ingredients and blend until smooth.

This will keep for up to 1 week in an airtight container in the fridge.

Apple Sauce

This makes a lovely topping for porridge, and goes great with granola and yoghurt. This will satisfy even the sweetest tooth.

500g apples
2 medjool dates
150ml water
1 tablespoon maple syrup
a pinch of ground cinnamon
    (optional)

Core the apples and chop into bite-size pieces (we prefer to leave the skin on our apples, as it contains most of the nutrition). Remove the stones from the dates.

Put into a saucepan with the rest of the ingredients, bring to the boil, then reduce the heat, put a lid on the pan and simmer gently for 20 minutes, stirring occasionally and checking to make sure there is enough water. The key to stewing fruit is to make sure you have enough water in the pan so that the fruit doesn't burn, and to keep the lid on to maintain the moisture, so add an extra splash of water if it's catching on the bottom of the pan.

When the apple has broken down and is completely tender, blend with a hand-held blender or in a blender or food processor until completely smooth.

This will keep for up to 1 week in an airtight container in the fridge.

Nutritional Information

All values per 100g

	Energy (kj)	Energy (kcal)	Fat	Fat (saturated)	Carbohydrates	Carbs (sugars)	Fibre	Protein	Salt
BREAKFAST									
Banoffee Overnight Oats 128	778	185	6.3g	1.9g	26g	14g	3.2g	4.4g	0.06g
Carrot Cake Chia Pudding 130	593	143	9.8g	5.1g	8.6g	6.2g	3.8g	3.2g	0.08g
PORRIDGE 3 WAYS 132									
Oat Groats 132	752	178	2.9g	0.6g	31g	4.6g	4.1g	4.8g	0.36g
Quick Easy Porridge 132	562	134	2.7g	0.4g	22g	2.9g	2.8g	3.9g	0.09g
3-grain Coconut Porridge 133	1,242	295	8.2g	5.1g	46g	2.2g	3.2g	8.2g	0.07g
Gluten-free Porridge Bread 134	1,142	273	13g	6.5g	29g	2.6g	3.5g	7.8g	1g
Fruit Compote *(Excluding the cinnamon)* 135	208	49	0.5g	0g	9.9g	9.4g	2.4g	0.8g	0g
Happy Gut 5-minute Berry Chia Jam 135	535	128	3.6g	0.4g	18g	16g	6.1g	2.4g	0g
Light Crunchy Granola 136	1,730	413	17g	6g	53g	13g	8.5g	8.7g	1.2g
Scrambled 'Eggs' on Toast 138 *(Excluding the toast)*	555	132	2.4g	0.6g	18g	1.5g	3.1g	7.9g	0.07g
SMOOTHIE BOWLS 3 WAYS 141									
Blueberry and Avocado 141	309	74	4g	0.8g	8g	5g	2.4g	1.5g	0.07g
Choc-oat-late Berry Bowl 141	461	110	4.5g	1.7g	11g	8.7g	5.4g	3.5g	004g
Pomegranate, Strawberries and Cream 141	433	104	6g	5.3g	9.2g	8.1g	1.7g	1.3g	0g
TOASTIE SPREADS 142									
Avocado, Tomato and Garlic 142	514	123	5g	1.2g	13g	2.5g	3.6g	3.7g	0.89g
Tahini, Banana and Cinnamon 142	946	225	8g	1.2g	28g	10g	5.3g	7.9	0.47g
Hummus, Miso and Cucumber 143	847	202	6.1g	0.9g	24g	2g	5.5g	9.8g	1.3g
Smoky Red Pepper Hummus, Sauerkraut, Cucumber 144	623	148	3.7g	0.5g	19g	2.3g	4.7g	6.9g	0.9g
Sweet Beet Hummus, Peanut Butter and Rocket 144	1,080	258	11g	2.4g	24g	3.1g	6.2g	12g	0.94g
Sweet Chocolate Treat 145 *(Includes 3g of goji berries)*	1,191	283	6.7g	2.8g	43g	25g	7.4g	8.6g	0.6g
Easy Strawberry Muffin 148 *(Using buckwheat flour)*	1,851	445	31g	3.4g	30g	13g	4.9g	8.8g	0.55g
Matcha and Buckwheat Almond Pancakes and Waffle 150	859	205	8.5g	0.8g	23g	8.2g	4.8g	6.3g	0.69g
Vegan Shakshuka 153 *(Excluding the avocado and anything to serve)*	213	51	1.3g	0.2g	5.3g	4.3g	1.8g	3.2g	0.5g
SOUP									
Thai Noodle Soup 156 *(Excluding any garnishes)*	713	170	6.8g	4.7g	20g	5.3g	2.9g	6g	0.83g

	Energy (kj)	Energy (kcal)	Fat	Fat (saturated)	Carbohydrates	Carbs (sugars)	Fibre	Protein	Salt
EASY MISO SOUP 3 WAYS *158*									
Summer veg *158*	266	63	1.2	0.2	5.9	2.3	3.1	5.7	4.2g
Spring veg *158*	550	131	4.4g	0.7g	8.7g	0.9g	3.9g	12g	4.3g
Winter veg *158*	397	94	1.1g	0.2g	13g	2.4g	3.9g	6.2g	4g
Lentil Sambar Soup *160* (Excluding the toasted seeds)	243	58	0.6g	0.1g	9.7g	2.7g	2.3g	2.2g	0.74g
Eat Your Greens Soup *163*	244	58	1.6g	1.2g	7.9g	1.5g	2.3g	1.8g	1g
Creamed Cauliflower and Coconut Soup *164*	337	80	3.2g	2.8g	10g	2.3g	1.7g	1.9g	0.6g
Maple Roasted Root Veg Soup *166* (Based on using vegetable stock and 1 teaspoon of salt)	271	64	0.5g	0g	13g	5.9g	2.5g	1.3g	0.54g
Sweet Potato and Chickpea Soup *167*	355	84	0.7g	0.1g	16g	4.3g	2.5g	2.2g	0.87g
SALADS									
Middle Eastern Greens Pot *170*	576	137	5.3g	0.7g	13g	2g	3.1g	7.4g	0.79g
Peanut Satay Tofu Pot *171*	767	184	9.7g	1.6g	11g	4.7g	3g	11g	1.3g
Japanese Teriyaki Tofu and Grain Bowl *174* (Using couscous)	754	180	8g	1.4g	15g	2.1g	4.1g	10g	0.98g
Lebanese Lemon Parsley Bean Salad *176* (Excluding any serving suggestions)	240	57	0.9g	0g	7.3g	1.9g	3g	3.2g	0.53g
Umami Greens and Noodle Salad *178*	489	116	3.3g	0.5g	15g	3.6g	2.5g	5.9g	1.5g
10-minute Creamy Bean and Grain Salad *180*	429	103	3.7g	1.8g	10g	3.1g	3.6g	4.6g	0.48g
Asian Broccoli Salad in a Sweet Smoky Chilli Sauce *181*	323	77	3.2g	0.4g	7.1g	5.4g	3.1g	3.4g	0.62g
Vegan Caesar Salad *182* (Based on the soy yoghurt dressing)	299	71	2.1g	0.4g	6g	2.9g	2.8g	5.3g	1.1g
Happy Gut High Protein Quinoa Salad *185*	498	227	11g	0.9g	22g	4.4g	4.3g	8.2g	1.1g
FANCIER LUNCHES									
Burrito Bowl *190*	350	83	2.1g	0.4g	11g	3.3g	3.4g	3.3g	0.42g
Vegan Hoisin 'Duck' Pancakes *192*	676	161	4.7g	0.7g	25g	13g	1.8g	4.2g	0.68g
FRITTERS 3 WAYS *194*									
Sweet Potato Fritters *194*	446	106	1.1g	0.2g	19g	4.4g	3.1g	3.7g	0.79g
Polish Potato Pancakes with Cannellini Beans (Placki Ziemniaczane) *195*	434	103	2.1g	0.2g	15g	1.8g	3.6g	3.9g	0.62g
Celeriac Bhajis *196*	548	130	2.1g	0.2g	18g	3g	5.1g	7.2g	1.6g
Toasted Wholemeal Pitta with Hummus, Rocket and Tomato (Without any extras) *198*	531	126	3.5g	0.4g	19g	2.8g	3g	3.3g	0.46g
Grilled Veggie and Tofu Kebabs with Chimichurri Sauce *199*	207	49	1.6g	0.2g	3.6g	2.1g	2g	4.1g	0.79g
Veggie Pot Noodle with Miso *200*	605	143	1.2g	0.2g	25g	3g	3.7g	5.9g	2.6g
QUICK EASIER DINNERS									
Easy Mexican Enchiladas *205*	674	161	6.3g	1.4g	18g	6.8g	3.6g	5.3g	1g
Creamy Spiced Black Bean Quesadillas *206*	911	218	12g	2.5g	17g	3.8g	4.1g	7.5g	0.57g
Easy Light Spicy Tacos *208*	441	105	3.4g	0.7g	14g	4.5g	4.4g	2g	0.39g
Pan-fried Tofu with Steamed Greens and Quinoa *210*	434	104	4.4g	0.7g	6.9g	1.9g	2g	8g	0.94g

	Energy (kj)	Energy (kcal)	Fat	Fat (saturated)	Carbohydrates	Carbs (sugars)	Fibre	Protein	Salt
Teriyaki Noodles *211*	425	101	1.3g	0.2g	17g	2.9g	2.2g	4.9g	1.4g
Japanese Veg and Noodle Ramen *212* (Including toppings, excluding any garnishes)	323	77	0.8g	0g	14g	3.8g	1.6g	3.3g	1.9g
Quick Burger *214*	543	129	2.7g	0.3g	17g	1.6g	4.3g	7.1g	1.1g
ONE POT DINNERS									
Vietnamese Coconut and Tempeh Curry *219*	497	119	4.1g	2.5g	13g	3.4g	3.1g	5.8g	1.1g
Low-FODMAP Malaysian Laksa Curry *220* (Using tofu and brown rice noodles)	737	176	7g	4.7g	21g	3.3g	2.5g	5.8g	1.2g
Humble Lentil Stew with Raita *221*	271	65	2.4g	1.8g	7.5g	3.3g	1.9g	2.2g	0.89g
Spinach and Butter Bean Curry *222*	250	60	2.6g	2.1g	5.2g	1.9g	2.4g	3g	0.52g
Jambalaya *224*	676	161	4.6g	1.4g	20g	2.4g	3.6g	7.6g	1.5g
Next Level Chilli Sin Carne *226*	310	74	3.8g	2.1g	6g	3.6g	3g	2.9g	0.58g
Spicy African Peanut Stew *227*	387	93	3.7g	0.8g	9.9g	3.3g	2.9g	3.8g	0.58g
Southern Indian Sweet Potato and Lentil Curry *228* (Excluding the pickled ginger)	417	99	3.2g	2.2g	12g	2.8g	2.7g	4.4g	0.61g
Tuscan Vegan Sausage and Bean Stew *230*	309	73	1.9g	0.6g	7.9g	3.2g	2.9g	4.8g	0.84g
PASTA DINNERS									
Easy Creamy Roasted Red Pepper Pasta *234*	588	140	4.3g	0.9g	18g	3.8g	3.2g	5.5g	0.97g
No Oil Creamy Carbonara *237*	658	156	3.3g	0.6g	22g	4.8g	4.7g	6.3g	1.2g
Spaghetti Bolognese *238*	398	94	0.5g	0g	18g	3.2g	1.5g	2.6g	0.68g
Creamy Broccoli and Mushroom Pasta Bake *239*	403	97	5.4g	0.7g	7.8g	0.9g	1.9g	3.4g	0.82g
No Oil Creamy Lasagna *242*	535	127	2.3	0.5	21	4.9	1.8	4.1	0.44
CENTREPIECE MEALS									
Cottage Pie with Sweet Potato Mash and Coriander Drizzle *246*	450	107	2.2g	0.4g	15g	2.7g	3g	5.3g	0.7g
Greek Spanakopita with Sweet Potato *248*	900	216	14g	5.3g	17g	2.5g	2.5g	5g	1.1g
Katsu Curry *251*	495	117	0.7g	0g	24g	3g	2.4g	2.7g	0.6g
SNACKS									
Kale Crisps *254*	349	83	1.7g	0.2g	3.8g	2.6g	5.4g	10g	3.2g
Happy Gut Hummus *256*	536	129	7.4g	1g	7.8g	0.5g	3.3g	5.9g	1.1g
Lower-in-fat Hummus 3 ways *256*	771	185	9.2g	1.2g	13g	1g	4.5g	9.5g	0.98g
Roasted Red Pepper Smoked Hummus *257*	664	159	7.6g	1g	13g	2.8g	4.5g	7.5g	0.81g
Sweet Beet Hummus *257*	655	157	7.5g	1g	12g	2.4g	4.6g	7.6g	0.84g
Buckwheat Flatbread *258* (Without additions)	1,548	366	2.9	0.6g	68g	2.5g	9.5g	12g	2.5g
Malted Yeast Bread *261*	1,437	340	1.8g	0.3g	64g	1.6g	8.5g	13g	2.2g
HEALTHIER DESSERTS									
Skinny Banana Bread *264*	877	207	1.3g	0.2g	45g	22g	2g	2.4g	0.84g

	Energy (kJ)	Energy (kcal)	Fat	Fat (saturated)	Carbohydrates	Carbs (sugars)	Fibre	Protein	Salt
ENERGY BALLS 2 WAYS *266*									
Tropical Energy Balls *266*	1,496	357	13g	6.4g	45g	27g	10g	8.8g	0.09g
Chocolate Hazelnut Delights *267*	1,460	348	12g	1.9g	49g	30g	7.8g	6.5g	0.13g
Healthier Hot Chocolate *268*	497	119	4.6g	1.2g	15g	11g	3.2g	2.5g	0.18g
Maple and Seed Flapjack *269*	2,161	520	36g	6.9g	36g	16g	7.2g	9.8g	0.09g
Berry Crumble *270* (Using frozen strawberries)	826	198	10g	4.8g	20g	12g	3.5g	4.3g	0g
4 SIMPLE HEALTHIER DESSERT SAUCES *272*									
Simple Date Caramel *272*	1,483	352	9.3g	0.8g	57g	56g	5.2g	6.9g	0.29g
Chocolate Sauce *272*	1,429	340	8.7g	2.4g	52g	51g	9.1g	7.6g	0.27g
Hazelnut Chocolate Spread *273*	1,386	332	18g	2.2g	33g	32g	5g	6.1g	0.2g
Apple Sauce *273*	345	81	0.5g	0g	18g	16g	1.5g	0.6g	0g

Index

Thanks

As we say in Ireland, 'thanks a million' for making it this far into our fifth book. We are still surprised to be called authors and we are chuffed to have been given the opportunity to try to inspire you to eat more veg and to understand some of the science behind the benefits of a plant-based diet.

Thanks to our families for supporting, inspiring and enriching our lives in so many ways. Thanks to Justyna, May, Theo and Ned; Sabrina, Elsie, Issy and Janet.

Special thanks to our Mom and Dad, Donal and Ismay, for without you both none of this would be possible. Thanks for the constant encouragement and inspiration and for always being there when we need support; Mom, thanks for caring so much and for always doing the less glamorous but vital jobs! Dad, thanks for always being there to advise and to guide us and The Happy Pear, we are eternally grateful.

Thanks to all the wonderful medical experts who we can now call friends who have contributed to this book and are such an important part of our courses. Firstly, massive thanks to Dr Alan Desmond. Thanks for being so up for life and for being such fun to work with and so incredibly professional as well. Al, your attention to detail and commitment is admirable. You've helped us so much with our courses and we are extremely grateful. Thanks to Rosie Martin for being a wonderful dietitian and a joy to work with – we love you, Rosie! Dr Sue, you're brilliant, so down-to-earth and relatable and also such a fountain of knowledge – it's really lovely to get to work with you. Thanks to Dr Gemma Newman, you're always so inspiring, lovely and we always love spending time with you. Thanks to Dr Joel Kahn – you're brilliant Joel, as well as being such an experienced cardiologist you're hilarious, real fun to work with and a total badass as well!

Massive thanks to our brothers Mark and Darragh. Darragh you are the unsung hero of The Happy Pear but so rarely get the recognition and limelight you deserve. We're very lucky to be your brothers. Mark, it's fabulous to have you back in the team colours! We're loving seeing you so much and working beside you again – thanks for being you, for being so straight, so cool and level-headed.

Thanks to Naomi Dooge for being an amazing home economist on this book and beyond; developing, testing, trialling and iterating recipes and ideas – thanks for being so wonderful to work with so closely, for being so professional as well as such a good wise friend over all these years. Thanks for putting up with our somewhat less structured approach to work and for being so good at what you do!

Seanie Cahill, thanks for the friendship. It's always wonderful to work with you – thanks for the inspiration, constant support and for always being there. Thanks for being so patient with us and for doing such a good job with all our videos!

Thanks to Paul Murphy for being such a vital part of The Happy Pear, for fitting in as though you were always a part of the HP and for being so wise considering your young age! Thanks for putting up with us all.